THE COMPLETE GUIDE TO PHYSICIAN RELATIONSHIPS

STRATEGIES FOR THE ACCOUNTABLE CARE ERA

KRISS BARLOW, RN, MBA

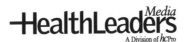

+HCPro

The Complete Guide to Physician Relationships: Strategies for the Accountable Care Era is published by HealthLeaders Media

ISBN: 978-1-60146-837-6

Kriss Barlow, RN, MBA, Author

Carrie Vaughan, Senior Editor

Bob Wertz, Executive Editor

Matt Cann, Group Publisher

Doug Ponte, Cover Designer

Mike Mirabello, Senior Graphic Artist

Lauren Rubenzahl, Proofreader

Matt Sharpe, Production Supervisor

Shane Katz, Art Director

Jean St. Pierre, Senior Director of Operations

Arrangements can be made for quantity discounts. For more information, contact:

HCPro, Inc.

75 Sylvan Street, Suite A-101

Danvers, MA 01923

Telephone: 800/650-6787 or 781/639-1872

Fax: 800/639-8511

E-mail: *customerservice@hcpro.com*

HCPro, Inc., is the parent company of HealthLeaders Media.

Visit HealthLeaders Media online at *www.healthleadersmedia.com*

Contents

       The Complete Guide to Physician Relationships

Chapter 7: What Do Physicians Want to Hear From Marketing?..........89

Chapter 8: Promoting Services 105

Chapter 9: Supporting Specialists 121

Chapter 10: What Do Physicians Want to Hear From Physician Relations?..........133

Contents

About the Author

Kriss Barlow, RN, MBA

Kriss Barlow, RN, MBA, has spent her entire professional career in the healthcare industry. Even at an early age, she witnessed hospital–physician communications through the eyes of her father, who was a physician.

Barlow holds a bachelor's degree in nursing from Augustana College and a master's degree in business administration from the University of Nebraska, and she has spent the past 15 years sharing her extensive knowledge of clinical and business development with clients and helping them with physician strategy—including relations, retention, sales, and medical staff development. Today, she is principal of Barlow/McCarthy, a consulting group focused on hospital–physician solutions. She focuses on strategy, communications, relationship, and retention models.

Although her clinical background helps in her current role, strategy, program development, and business solutions are her real passions. She treasures the chance to work with so many healthcare professionals and the opportunity to help them achieve success.

A recognized expert, Barlow is a frequent speaker whose presentations are full of content collected through her vast experiences in the healthcare industry and made more lively by her many stories from the hospital trenches. She frequently presents at the Forum for Healthcare Strategists, the Society for Healthcare Strategy and Market Development of the American Hospital Association, The American Association of Physician Liaisons, and numerous state and local conferences. Barlow is a frequent speaker for HealthLeaders Media's webcasts. She is a faculty member for the American Academy of Medical Management's Physician Recruitment program and serves on the Board of Directors for the National Medical Staff Certification program. She is also a certified sales instructor.

Barlow is the author of the HealthLeaders Media book, *A Marketer's Guide to Physician Relations*, and coauthor of a previous book, *Physician Relations Today: A Model for Growth*.

When she isn't working, it is all about family. Her husband Doug is the steadying force in her life and her biggest supporter. Together, they have three fabulous sons, two charming daughters-in-law, and a couple of adorable grandchildren. With one of her "boys" in the middle of an orthopedic residency, the cycle of medical staff relationships has taken on a personal feel.

Acknowledgments

The idea for this book was mine, but the interest and willpower to make it happen came from many fabulous people. It's because of them that I completed the physician surveys for this book and the content came together in a meaningful way.

To accomplish the surveys, I called on friends and colleagues in physician relations, marketing, and leadership roles across the country. Here's a huge shout-out and note of gratitude to all the physician relations reps who carried the survey to their practices and assisted in getting a strong survey response. It was a huge favor to ask, and I am grateful to each and every person who participated.

The topic of physician communication is front and center in the minds of our clients, and I tapped many of them to share a thought or offer insight. They are the innovators who consistently strive to enhance the experience for their doctors and their teams. It was an honor to work with such talented professionals.

The team at Barlow/McCarthy went above and beyond. I am proud to be associated with each of them. Allison McCarthy, Ann Maloley, and Michael Barber, MD, offered expertise and words of wisdom in those topic areas where they are experts; you'll see their content in the chapters. Ann did double duty, proofing the content to keep me on track. Dave Zirkle, PhD, lives in the world of analytics and survey work; he kept me on track with the data elements. I am proud of the team and the work they do to help each other and to make a difference for our clients.

On a personal note, the center of my ability to work passionately in this field is my husband, Doug, and our boys. From the bottom of my heart, I thank my family for their love and support. It enables me to freely grow in my profession.

Introduction

True confession: I love healthcare. I passionately believe in the commitment to healing and appreciate that every day the people in healthcare make a difference in the lives of others. I am proud to say this is my field of choice. I am surrounded by good people doing great work and, yet, communication within the healthcare ranks is not all it could or should be. That's what drives me and why I initiated this effort. I firmly believe that it's important to know how we can better understand the needs of our key stakeholder group: physicians.

Why This Topic?

I am frequently asked, "What do you find to be the most effective way to communicate with physicians?" And even though weekly conversations with doctors give me a sense of what works—and a better sense of what doesn't work—I always feel a little uncertain about being the expert opinion on this. We've all heard the advertising rule that messages need to be repeated up to seven times to be heard. But will doctors really tolerate that much repetition? There must be a way to communicate with physicians that is more efficient not only for the communicators but for the physicians as well.

In our message-filled lives, there is so much determination to get through and find innovative ways to ensure that our words are the ones that get heard through all the clutter. Yet we often wonder about the keys to effective communication. Is it how the content is shared, the message itself, or the circumstances of our environment that impact our listening? It is probably a bit of each. But when it comes to connecting with physicians, seasoned healthcare professionals want to make the message meaningful and relevant. We don't get many chances, and it is often information that we need them to have, so we want to make the process efficient and desirable.

Healthcare organizations are looking for ways to align more closely with physicians, which means it is even more important to find out how physicians like messages to be delivered and what they believe to be most important. This book is the result of asking those types of questions—190 doctors shared their opinions in response to questions in four areas of interest. We asked what they want to hear from healthcare leaders, from marketing, from physician relations, and from their peers—especially as it relates to referral relationships. (Full details of the research respondents and methodology are in the appendix.)

The Content

Getting input straight from the source always raises awareness. We can no longer say, "That's just Dr. Whiner, he always has something negative to say." The result of research is that we see trends without names, which provides a less biased view of the issue. It also gives us a chance to revisit our personal perspectives on the topic.

- Common wisdom is that it's always best to get answers "straight from the horse's mouth." So in order to understand the best method of

The Complete Guide to Physician Relationships

communication and most meaningful content for doctors, we asked physicians. If the responses varied based on demographic or specialty differences, we called those out in the text. Interestingly, there was a great deal of consistency in the top responses.

- While leadership teams will likely want to explore the implications of the survey findings alongside their strategy, we do offer tactical suggestions that can help jump start the implementation.

- In addition, perspectives and suggestions from market leaders are provided throughout the book. Our industry colleagues are always anxious to hear how others are approaching a topic. Market leaders have weighed in with opinions about the survey findings and their recommendations.

There's a lot of theory out there about communications, and much of it is fabulous reading. With all that we hope the book can be, however, it is not going to provide that. The intent of this book is to provide data to help us define our methods and messages to enhance success and push communication to drive measurable benefits as we work with our physician audience.

What Do Physicians Want to Hear From Leadership?

"The art of communication is the language of leadership."
—James Humes

There are many references about the relationship between organizational leaders and physicians in healthcare publications, in webinars, and on the speaking circuit. We get it! There is a need for healthcare organizations and their leadership to be in sync with the medical staff. Leaders are acutely aware of the need to balance cost containment and care delivery. In the *2011 HealthLeaders Media Industry Survey,* cost reduction was the highest priority for leaders, with 35% selecting it as one of their top three priorities—quality/patient safety ran a close second, at 33%. Care delivery is at the center of our discussions, but collaboration to manage cost effectiveness is the driver. And although models and methods abound, at the heart of change is the ability to talk with each other—the need to appreciate the business and personal challenges of each party.

Physicians still have room for improvement with their ability to listen to other perspectives and give leaders who are trying a chance. But building that trust is tough to do in the healthcare market. This survey is not about acknowledging trust issues or calling out what the physicians should do differently; rather, it is about providing leaders insight into what the physicians want to hear.

The data highlights priorities for the future success of leaders and the physicians they work with and also provides perceptions about organizational cultures and perspectives. As we anticipate closer working relationships between physicians and healthcare organizations, it is key to understand where doctors believe the organization does an excellent job and where healthcare organizations do not perform as well. The survey was designed to understand how well physicians believe their organization does in several key areas. Other survey questions centered on physicians' views of where leaders need to focus their attention for the medical staff and, more specifically, what aspect of the new hospital–physician relationship is most important to them. Not surprisingly, the desire for involvement—control—of one's own destiny is apparent in the survey results.

Remember that the survey was implemented to expose communications, so as we discuss operational challenges or business structures, the intent is not to build out the method, only to define and then detail what they want to hear—with a little bit of when and how.

Where the Medical Staff Wants Support From Hospital Leaders

The survey respondents can be grouped almost equally into two categories
(see Figure 1.1):

- Those who want healthcare leaders focused on care delivery

- Those who desire attention on the business relationships

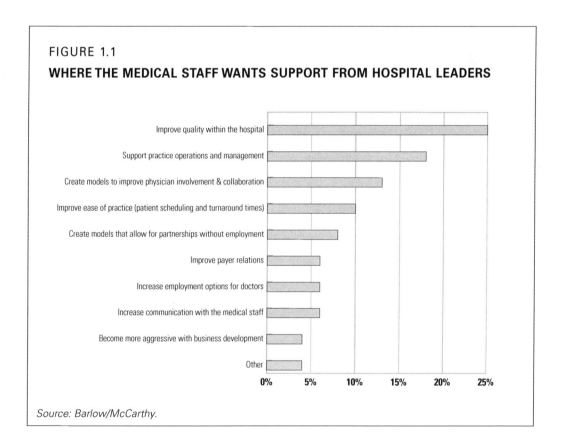

FIGURE 1.1

WHERE THE MEDICAL STAFF WANTS SUPPORT FROM HOSPITAL LEADERS

Source: Barlow/McCarthy.

Twenty-five percent of respondents say quality is the most important obligation of leadership over the next three years. This would indicate that doctors are listening to health reform messages on the topic of quality and collaboration, as well as having a strong desire to provide good care to their patients. An additional 13% felt that the leaders' most important role was to improve physician involvement and collaboration. Another category that emerged as a priority under the umbrella of hospital operations was the need to make it easier to practice at the facility, which scored 10%. In total, 48% responded that the focus should be on the care delivery side of the equation.

None of the collaborative business/practice strategies scored very high as a standalone, but when grouped together, 36% of the respondents say these strategies are their single choice for hospital leadership's support of the medical staff. It included a small number (6%) who want increased employment, almost 18% of physicians who want practice support, 8% who desire partnerships without employment, and 4% who cited more aggressive business development.

In the "other" category, respondents most frequently mentioned physician recruitment. (You will see this topic called out later in the survey as well.)

For most of the survey questions, there was more unity around the answers than for this one. The differences may be due to the level of in-hospital involvement, so we evaluated the data by primary care physicians (PCP) vs. specialists:

- Improving quality is the most important element to both PCPs and specialists; however, is it emphasized more by specialists

- PCPs are more likely to identify practice management/support than specialists

The Complete Guide to Physician Relationships

When survey respondents were asked to select one answer, 5% chose multiple answers—which may say something about their perception that one priority is not enough.

Priorities and agendas

Today's leaders have a lot going on. As they evaluate medical staff relationships with clinical, business, and peer groups, multiple obligations are in play. The physicians responding in this survey are almost equally divided on their perceptions of the leader's priority to support the medical staff. At face value, it leaves strong leadership teams challenged to determine what to tackle first. And this is only the medical staff's agenda—there are others, of course.

Getting the local pulse

There are national trends and then local realities. With regard to the priorities and expectations of your local medical staff, it's imperative to dig deeper into their needs, the pulse of the local market, and the priorities. Starting with data, the decision support team can assist the leadership in understanding which physicians fall into that "can't afford to lose" category. Use the data to first project their three-year practice plan. You can use data like age, admissions patterns, and tenure with the organization, as well as qualitative details like recent discussions regarding employment or group merger to get a sense of their ability to remain in this category.

Next, carve out those physicians that you perceive to be future leaders. You may find some in the "can't afford to lose" category, whereas others may be active in practice building and may be splitting current referrals. Focus on these two categories first. Leaders should meet personally with these doctors—there will be a time for group discussion (primarily for action and implementation) later. If your organization has leaders who have been engaging with medical staff on a regular basis, use that group. If the physician relations team has a strong relationship with the doctors who have been selected, then ask them to facilitate the discussion with leadership.

The personal meeting has value at several levels. First, you are able to clearly discern the priorities of your vital medical staff members. Second, it sets the stage for shared development. And third, it is a proactive method of reaching in and framing a model for ongoing communication.

Even though some CEOs may say it is too time-consuming, if it is staged and well coordinated, it can actually be a time saver. Instead of fighting the rumor mill, create the message.

Quality

As it does in many conversations with physicians about priorities in today's healthcare environment, quality bubbled at the top in this study as well. The physicians' responses to having leaders focus on quality improvement likely leaves some leaders saying, "They have no idea about all the quality work we are doing." Physicians clearly want the hospital to exceed expectations in quality and to create a safer and better experience for themselves and their patients.

Whereas leaders recognize all of the efforts internally to enhance quality within the hospital, physicians recognize only those elements that impact them on a personal level. The gap between these two areas may fall to directors and managers to regularly remind the doctors of the strides that have been made to work on quality and to share the information in a way that is patient care–centric. Data can be shared that graphically shows the impact of quality initiatives. Physicians can be asked to weigh in on quality initiatives that will impact them. Rather than creating a committee, consider a meeting or a task force that includes two sessions with very actionable agendas and outcomes. The beauty of their desire for quality is that everyone wants the same end result, and the language of data speaks for both parties.

Support at the practice level

Second to quality, getting the hospital's support in practice operations and management is on the minds of physicians, with almost 18% of survey respondents indicating so. This is great news for hospital leaders in that physician practices view the hospital as a resource for more support and are willing to ask for it. For those physicians who want more support, there is the challenge of practice management in a tough economic climate with more change to come. Organizations should define where are the opportunities to help physicians—for example, by evaluating the type of tools that could be offered and the fit of those tools with what the doctors in your market desire.

Best practice in this area would be to make sure that you only offer what you know you can deliver. And let doctors' needs be the driver of your actions. Resist the temptation to create practice support strategies that are more focused on what you need them to do to help you grow your business. If you stay focused on their practice development needs, you'll gain in the long run. Careful messaging for your team around what can be done legally and what should be done politically will of course make for an appreciated value-add.

Beyond Doing, Communicating

Each week, I see organizations and leaders doing great things. There is a great deal of time, energy, and money spent on trying to enhance the physician experience, the communication flow, and providing a service that will add value for the physicians and their patients. But the sad reality is that many doctors really don't see it, feel it, or appreciate it.

Even as an outsider, that is frustrating; however, it is a problem that can be solved. Physicians will rarely initiate a strategic discussion. Communication with leaders is generally around tactical needs, personal agenda items, or issues that need to be resolved. Most leaders focus on strategy and prefer to be in the future tense rather than the daily issues. Proactive communication about strategy that has value for the physician must be leader-initiated. Sometimes this starts with involvement in the strategic plan; for other organizations, it can be around a physician partnership model; still others use national leadership conferences or local classes to immerse the right group of physicians in understanding of strategy.

By understanding strategy, communication about setting and reaching goals sets the stage for enhanced communication. Physicians rarely want to be told the final outcome; rather, give them the tools to experience how it was determined.

SPEAK MY LANGUAGE

Consider how physicians learn. Most physicians have undergraduate degrees in science; their advanced training was about deductive reasoning and ruling out conditions. And their practice success is based on an ability to determine what is wrong. Understanding the choices, the rationale, and the process is comfortable for them. When a solution is provided without an understanding of how it was derived, the result is often doctors questioning, second-guessing, and needing to work through the detail. Why not present the process and approach, then the outcome?

Getting the clinical house in order

Physicians who have practices with heavy hospital patient volume have increasingly called out the importance of quality. It is not a stretch to say that every hospital is working on quality initiatives; however, the level of physician engagement in the processes is variable. It is important to encourage early physician involvement. Hospitals struggle to enforce quality processes without physician buy-in, and buy-in will not occur without involvement. Shared quality goals need to be just that: nurses and doctors working together with leaders supporting the process to discern the obligations for every party. So, we are back to communication again.

As organizations work to do more with less, to better manage costs, and to improve quality, success will depend on tighter alignment and shared goals. Everyone in the system wants to do the right thing for the patient. In many decision points—including scheduling and operational processes—there is more than one way. Involve doctors, consider options, and be open to change about the process.

We have all heard the analogy of herding cats as we try to get physicians to align. As the clinical process is enhanced through physician involvement, the best communication to other physicians often comes from one of their own. Growing physician leaders is absolutely essential, and this is a great place to message from within the physician community.

INSIDER'S VIEW

SHIFTING MODELS OF CARE

Amy Dirks Stevens, regional vice president, strategy & business development/CSO at Provena Health, shared her thoughts on this portion of the survey data. In the old hospital–physician relationship model, she says to physicians, hospitals looked frustratingly similar to their noncompliant patients. "We asked for help, but didn't consistently follow our physicians' advice. We wanted to get a clear diagnosis, unless the treatment required change. It would probably take a crisis to motivate us to real action. We needed our doctor, far more than our doctor needed us."

Now, there's a shift, Stevens says. "Physicians and hospitals need the best shared continuum of quality to even remain on payer panels. With their larger scale, hospitals are becoming natural aggregators of 'back office' services to reduce the burden of practice management, whether the physician is employed or independent. And both hospitals and physicians are creating new business models that share the risk of income tied to outcomes."

Today's version of alignment isn't about improving "poor medical staff communications." In fact, if we're honest, there will be many physicians and hospitals left behind who simply won't meet the higher thresholds that will be expected of us. Alignment, this time, is about tangible business integration aimed at preserving financial viability while improving quality of care.

Business Models

Employment

National data tells us that organizations expect to grow the number of employed physicians. The September 2010 *HealthLeaders Media Intelligence Unit* report, "Physician Alignment in an Era of Change" concluded that at present, 16% of physicians are hospital employed, but 74% of hospitals are planning to employ more physicians in the next one to three years. Of interest is that 70% of hospitals report increased requests for employment by physicians, and half of physicians completing residencies are now hospital employed.

Employment is a viable business model. Primary care employment has been a key strategy in many markets for years. Specialty referrals are very common when smaller markets don't have depth in specialists, and hospitals have used employment as a strategy to shore up a market and protect some ancillary income.

Organizations feel they have done a good job of communicating their employment strategy with their medical staff. Perhaps that is the reason they did not earn a higher score on this survey. The physicians are aware of the employment strategy, and those who wish to opt for employment are in conversations or have signed the contract.

The right type of partnerships

With so many options beyond employment, like management and comanagement agreements, joint ventures, gain sharing models, medical staff offices, or California's Foundation models, leaders are striving to find the "best one" and to make certain that their interests are represented. I asked Richard Keck, founder and president of StratEx, to address the topic of partnerships and whether there is a perfect—or near perfect—business partnership for hospitals and physicians at this time.

Keck says that structure follows strategy. Partnerships are formed to accomplish specific goals or tasks. Whether it is reducing infection rates or building a free-standing ambulatory care center, they are the legal and organizational structures that enable hospitals and physicians to work together to accomplish specific goals.

> *"The most important aspect of partnerships*
> *are the mutual goals of the respective parties."*
> —*Richard Keck*

The foundation for successful partnerships are agreed-upon measurable goals/outcomes and a plan to accomplish those goals that includes a financial projection. This helps ensure that the parties are clear about what they are trying to accomplish and the anticipated outcomes, thereby increasing chances for success. Plans are obsolete the moment they are published, but they do provide understanding of the implications of variations in revenue or expenses, so the parties can make the necessary adjustments to meet their mutual goals.

The regulations defining hospital–physician partnerships are constantly changing. Once the parties have agreed upon mutual goals and a business plan, a partnership agreement should be drafted with the help of legal counsel and other experts. Make sure that communication about this process is shared with the doctors and that there is recognition about who, what, and when. Waiting can breed nervousness.

Whether the partnerships are structured employment contracts, joint ventures, consulting agreements, or the latest legal structure, they are all reduced to a written agreement between the two parties that identify a set of mutual goals and commitments. Partnerships are about accomplishing specific goals. Legal and organizational structures are the enablers, *not* the drivers.

Before the contract is signed, physicians and the organization need to understand their obligations at a very tactical level. This includes team building, quality obligations, performance expectations, and, yes, communication expectations.

BASIC CONSIDERATIONS

- Create a planned approach to earn trust postcontract. Assumptions about this will backfire every time.

- Under promise, over deliver. Keep track of what is delivered. Communicate this verbally and often—it needs to be in writing.

- Plan regular, face-to-face meetings for the first six months to review what was promised on both sides and what is being delivered, on both sides.

- Do not delegate all the communication to others. If it is the leader's vision to have the partnership in place, then the leader needs to stay engaged in the early implementation.

Several of these emerging business models will further push organization leaders and physicians together, says Keck. Business and financial decisions take center stage when the two parties discuss a more formal relationship. Leaders should plan for implementation specifics and obligations in advance. Challenges with the relationships, obligations, and communication may rear their heads after the two parties seal the deal.

One size never fits all

It is fascinating to observe market response and market sensitivity as different models are considered. The domino effect has long been observed with regard to employment of physicians. By market, when a few groups go, then many others follow. It seems like a permission thing—once a prestigious medical group opts into the business arrangement, others have the freedom to follow. For others, chronic financial challenges are a part of the equation. And for the doctor just finishing residency or fellowship, debt load and job security are front and center.

Payer ranks low—a no control issue?

Because this was a priority for less than 6% of the physician's surveyed, it may fall into the category of one of many important things, but not the most important for the majority of those surveyed. Is it safe to assume that the private practices have payer strategies in place, such as deciding which payer groups they want on their roster, and employed physicians have this managed by the employing entity? This area will likely get more complicated as a result of health reform.

Real Involvement

It is interesting to note that 12% of the survey respondents believe the number one leadership need is physician involvement and collaboration. At a time when many are feeling pulled in every direction, a small percentage of doctors want this to happen above all other leadership priorities for working with the medical staff. But does this mean they are enlightened or concerned?

If you ask, then listen, and make sure that they do, too

When asked to interview members of the medical staff, some of the messages I hear seem to be repeated regardless of geography or organization size. One is, "Now they have hired someone to hear the same message I have told them." If I heard it once, it would not have had impact, but I actually hear this more than half of the time. Where is the communication breakdown? Is it a lack of listening, a lack of responding to the suggestion, or not doing anything about it—either because the organization can't or shouldn't?

On the flip side, maybe a reply was given to the doctors and they were not listening. The starting point is to really understand what was shared. If the request is outrageous or illegal, say so right away. If it is a fair request but you cannot address it, then promptly say so, verbally and in writing, along with rationale for why not. If there are alternatives, give them.

Physician surveys are an excellent way to gather suggestions or concerns en masse. The results allow you to understand the priorities and gauge the time frame and approach for responding. It is a great way to understand topics of interest for communication. Once a survey has been evaluated, a solid approach for communicating the actions is in order. The following is an example of one option:

- Those who participated are thanked. A plan of action is detailed. Some medical staffs do not appreciate the length of time it takes to get the survey processed and to receive the report; let them know.

- When ready, a short list of priority actions needs to be communicated to medical staff leaders. They can suggest other medical staff members who may be interested in supporting the change.

- Communicate the first list of priorities in committees and through communication tools. Make sure that the message is brief and shows action and timelines.

- Once the suggestion is implemented, remind the medical staff of their request and the action. If you have a physician relations team, ask them to remind the medical staff again at year-end.

- Prepare a fair and balanced response to the expressed suggestions and needs that cannot be met. It's important to acknowledge them and give rational reasons why they can't happen.

It's important to note that you should only do physician surveys if your organization is in a position to react or respond to them. For example, if your organization has been jolted by a new market dynamic or an aggressive competitor, take the time you need to get that in order before you start asking physicians to add to your already full plate of priorities that you may not have the time or resources to address. But because we're talking about communication, it's important to note here that, even in this case, the physicians should be involved.

The slow 'no' is detrimental

When physicians have ideas for growing their service, or improving the service, the typical approach was to take this information to a service leader or member of the C-suite. The usual result is that they would generally get an update about the capital budget expenditures, time frames, and priorities and be told by the leader, "We'll get back to you." Some leaders pride themselves on their ability to implement the slow no as a way to manage the medical staff. This approach erodes relationships at a time when they are already a bit suspect.

Do you remember hearing the quote by General Colin Powell, "The day soldiers stop bringing you their problems is the day you have stopped leading them"? It goes without saying that the magnitude of pain grows when there is a sense that decisions were made without input or the decision was made but not shared. In the past decade, many believed that a good CEO was able to share "just enough." In some schools, there is still a bit of this old thinking, and it is hurting communication at every level.

Summary

All successful partnerships are based on mutual respect and trust. Trust and mistrust are learned behaviors. One of the keys to establishing trust in effective hospital–physician communication is consistency and transparency. The structure of the healthcare system is increasingly putting hospitals and physicians into adversarial positions—usually around money.

A leader's trust with the medical staff is built on predictability and transparency. Although both parties have work to do around these principles, hospitals have the greatest burden. Lack of accurate, timely, and consistent information is one of the big drivers of mistrust between hospitals and physicians. Hospitals must do a better job not only with their physicians but also with their staff and the public. Physicians are scientists—their currency is timely, accurate, and reliable information.

The survey shares where the medical staff believes leaders should focus. This paves the way for conversation and opportunity.

How Does Your Hospital Compete?

Physicians ranked their organization's ability to compete on quality, medical staff, nursing quality, patient satisfaction, technology, cost, physician recruitment, and retention fairly well across the board (see Figure 2.1). By school grading standards, every area received passing grades of B+ to C+. Their organization's ability to compete in quality received top marks, with a score of 4.41 out of 5, or an 88%. Medical staff quality was next with a score of 4.36, or 87%. This aligns with results of other surveys that show physicians usually state that their own quality and capabilities are key contributors to the organization's success.

Nursing quality, patient satisfaction, and technology also scored better than 4 out of 5. The two areas that received the lowest scores are cost and physician recruitment and retention at 3.8 out of 5. In the area of cost, with so much pressure on practices to cut corners, it is likely they evaluated how well their hospital partners are working through that process with them. Many hospitals have asked physicians to make changes in procedures, equipment, and practice routines to help better manage those costs. What we don't know from the survey is how involved the physicians have been in cost-cutting measures at the hospital level. If the physicians think, for example, that other choices could have been considered to streamline costs but they weren't consulted, it may have impacted the ranking.

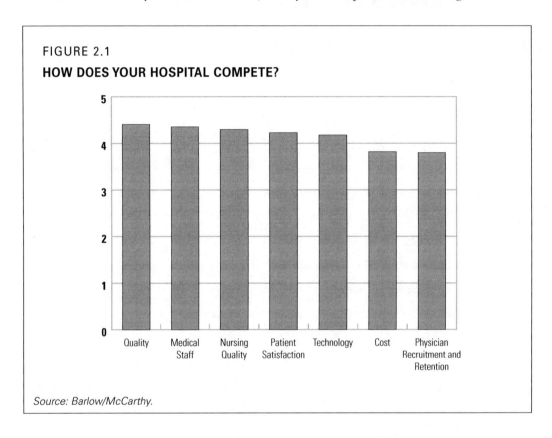

FIGURE 2.1

HOW DOES YOUR HOSPITAL COMPETE?

Source: Barlow/McCarthy.

The lowest score is physician recruitment and retention. There may have been multiple factors at play here, including personal experience with needing to recruit or seeing a colleague leave.

          The Complete Guide to Physician Relationships

As part of our data analysis, we looked at the survey results by subset to discern any appreciable differences. In most other questions of this study, the replies were fairly consistent regardless of age, type of practice, or location. However, replies did vary by age for this question (see Figure 2.2).

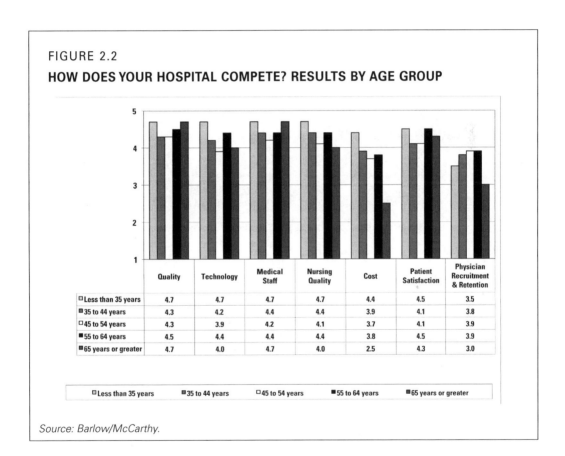

FIGURE 2.2

HOW DOES YOUR HOSPITAL COMPETE? RESULTS BY AGE GROUP

	Quality	Technology	Medical Staff	Nursing Quality	Cost	Patient Satisfaction	Physician Recruitment & Retention
Less than 35 years	4.7	4.7	4.7	4.7	4.4	4.5	3.5
35 to 44 years	4.3	4.2	4.4	4.4	3.9	4.1	3.8
45 to 54 years	4.3	3.9	4.2	4.1	3.7	4.1	3.9
55 to 64 years	4.5	4.4	4.4	4.4	3.8	4.5	3.9
65 years or greater	4.7	4.0	4.7	4.0	2.5	4.3	3.0

Less than 35 years   35 to 44 years   45 to 54 years   55 to 64 years   65 years or greater

Source: Barlow/McCarthy.

The youngest segment of physicians was the most positive, giving higher scores in every category—except recruitment and retention—than their peers.

The oldest group (over the age of 65) appears more negative on many items, although they tend to rank their organization's ability to compete the highest in those areas that they believe physicians more closely impact, such as medical staff and quality. This group also rated the organization's ability to compete on cost and physician recruitment at the lowest level of any other age group.

Conversations About Cost, Technology

Leaders in the various organizations that I work with have a really good sense of the fiscal responsibilities of the entity. They understand finance and the business side of running an organization, including areas that make money and areas that serve the population but at an expense to the system. Healthcare leaders ranked cost reduction first as an area of focus in the next three years in the *2011 Health-Leaders Media Industry Survey*, so it is clearly a priority. Unfortunately, leaders may not be communicating the organization's efforts and earning the physicians' commitment to follow suit at the hospital.

> *"Physicians are critical to the success of quality initiatives in healthcare.*
> *While many times, quality and cost may be aligned, physicians*
> *do not always see this. As leaders, we need to engage them more in our*
> *quality and seek to better understand their thoughts on cost."*
> *—Marian M. Furlong, president and CEO of Hudson Hospital & Clinics*

The Complete Guide to Physician Relationships

Management team owns communication about cost

Although top-level leaders do a nice job of talking about costs with doctors, they simply cannot carry the message alone—nor should they. It is about securing buy-in at the level closest to the experience. Directors and managers are much closer to the experience and are in a position to have frequent exchanges with physicians at a very tangible cost level. Leaders should educate their management team at this level. Once the management feels comfortable with cost realities, they should be obligated to show, tell, and talk about efforts to streamline cost with doctors. The following are tips to improve communication about costs with doctors:

- Encourage management to understand cost containment at a conversational level to communicate more effectively with staff, other executives, and physicians.

- Solicit feedback from physicians on potential areas of waste within the health system. It may not make a huge impact, but it is one way to engage them in a positive way. If they want to contribute here, let them.

- Show physicians the numbers. In clinical areas where there is documented need to streamline costs, physicians would benefit from seeing all the actions in play, with the numbers, rather than being told about the single area of cost reduction that they are being asked to implement.

Hospital does not equal small business

Beyond engaging and enlightening the staff and physicians about specifics of cost containment, a dose of reality about the budgetary challenges of running a hospital is also a good thing to share. A hospital is much different to run than a practice. There are expenses and obligations that are just a part of doing business. Look at those areas that will be relevant and of interest for your doctors. Help them see how physicians can impact—positively or negatively—the hospital's financials. If your organization has physicians who grouse about this topic, and you believe they are truly interested, ask your CFO to create a presentation that calls out some of the rules and financial obligations.

Talking about money will be front and center in the accountable care organization conversations, so it is even more important now to find a place to start that earns credibility about financial dealings before it is their money we're talking about.

Technology is often personal

There is the ongoing dichotomy between the organization's need to cut costs and the need to stay competitive with clinical technology. And we know this technology costs money. This push/pull dilemma makes open, balanced communication between physicians and clinical leaders even more necessary.

In the survey group, 7% scored technology a 2—that's a D in letter grades. I suspect that if we pulled out the individual surveys for those physicians, it would be individuals that need technology to differentiate their expertise and/or those who are up against competing facilities that have all the bells and whistles.

It's fair to say that technology can help build an organization's brand in highly competitive markets, so physicians should have a voice on this topic. If they have the clinical expertise, they'll want the technology to match their ability. This goes a long way in physician satisfaction and can ultimately help drive business.

As we focus on leaders communicating with physicians about this topic, we'd like to say, "Give them what they want," but we know that is not always realistic or feasible. What shouldn't happen is letting the doctor believe he will get the desired technology and then not delivering it. Leaders should determine whether the managers and directors who need to communicate this information are trained to give the right message. Physicians often tell me, "It's not the director—he wanted to get this for me. The 'higher ups' were the ones who slashed it from the budget." That certainly does not earn credibility for top level leaders. Anyone who needs to deliver messages about equipment/technology requests that are denied will benefit from coaching. Nobody means to throw the other party under the bus, but in this area, it happens very frequently.

Patient Satisfaction

Physicians participating in the survey gave a lukewarm level of confidence in their organization's ability to compete on patient satisfaction. I asked Kristin Baird, RN, BSN, MHA, president and CEO of Baird Group and a national expert in patient experience, what factors may be behind these survey results. This response may reflect that physicians aren't aware of, or engaged in, patient satisfaction improvement efforts that are underway, she says. Many, if not most, healthcare organizations are measuring patient satisfaction and making efforts at improvement through customer service strategies and training but aren't including the medical staff, Baird explains. "Up until a few years ago, many providers fell somewhere between oblivious and unconcerned with patient satisfaction scores. *Hospital Consumer Assessment of Healthcare Providers and Systems* have placed patient satisfaction scores squarely in the public eye, leaving little doubt about its importance. The era of consumer-driven healthcare, fueled by transparency has given new focus to patient satisfaction. Healthcare organizations that don't engage the physicians in the quest for service excellence are missing a great opportunity."

HOW TO ENGAGE PHYSICIANS IN PATIENT SATISFACTION EFFORTS

Kristin Baird shares four strategies that healthcare leaders can follow to engage physicians in patient satisfaction improvement efforts.

1. Inform

  • Keep patient satisfaction scores front and center, reminding physicians that the scores represent the voice of their patients

  • Educate physicians on *Hospital Consumer Assessment of Healthcare Providers and Systems* (HCAHPS) and the link to reimbursement

  • Let physicians know about service improvement initiatives that are underway and encourage them to get involved

2. Include

  • Make physicians part of action teams

  • Solicit their input about how to make improvements

3. Inspire

  • Connect service initiative to the mission, vision, and values

  • Share stories about great service with the medical staff as well as with those on the front lines

4. Identify best practices and superstars

  • Like everyone else, physicians deserve recognition for going above and beyond in serving their patients, yet they are often left out of formal recognition efforts

The best practices in the industry are those that have physicians who are actively engaged in improving the patient experience, says Baird. "They have a strong service champion in medical staff leadership and set clear standards for physicians as well as front line staff. Unfortunately, many organizations shy away from including physicians in service improvement initiatives."

In order to get the physicians engaged in service improvement, it's necessary to show the business case for a great patient experience, supported by data and punctuated with patient stories that will resonate. The combination of data and stories engages the head and the heart. At the same time, it's important to share information about what actions are underway to make improvements.

Some organizations have tied monetary incentives for physicians to improve patient satisfaction, Baird says. "I'm not certain that this has been effective. I just don't know. But to me, it makes perfect sense. There is no hesitation about incentivizing productivity. Isn't the patient experience just as important as volume to the organization's financial well-being? It's important for the physicians to understand that productivity and patient satisfaction are not mutually exclusive. You can achieve both quite successfully, so why not include both in a balanced scorecard?"

No one argues that clinical quality is an imperative. But quality (as defined by the patient) is in the eye of the beholder. Patients are more likely to judge quality on their experience. This comes down to their perceptions of how well they were treated by the staff and physicians. When presented with data alone, many physicians will argue about the validity and reliability of the data. But, when paired with qualitative research such as focus groups or mystery shopping, many physicians will begin to accept the need to change things. I've seen physicians do a complete 180 after observing focus groups or reading a mystery shopper report where patients tell their stories about horrendous experiences with their medical practice. Qualitative information moves the information from the head to the heart. And that's when real change happens.

Recruitment and Retention

The research findings suggest that physicians perceive their organizations could improve their ability to recruit and retain physicians, says Allison McCarthy, principal at Barlow/McCarthy and a recognized recruitment expert who works closely with senior executives and in-house recruiters. The competitive intensity around physician supply/demand means the passive approaches of the past no longer work. Whether it is trying to recruit into their own practice or observing their hospital trying to do the same on their behalf, the days of being able to simply "make a few calls" or "place an ad" and generate several qualified candidates have fallen by the wayside.

Today's competition for physician talent translates into lots of options and choice for those seeking a new practice opportunity. They look for the situation that will best meet their needs—personal and professional. If they make a mistake and accept the wrong position, they just leave for something else.

A change in approach is needed to successfully recruit physicians today, including the following.

The Complete Guide to Physician Relationships

- Defining the practice opportunity with an "outside in" perspective. With lots of practice options available to recruits, what you have to offer must be translated into what they want and need—personally and professionally (i.e., the type of care to be provided [maximize their expertise], the ability to grow a successful practice [referral sources], and recognition as a vital member of the provider community).

- Ensuring recruitment readiness by having a sound business plan in place, confirming medical staff support, demonstrating the desire to recruit in both words and actions, and providing enough capital (financial and human resource) to deliver on promises made during the search.

- Proactive efforts that are both short- and long-term in focus. Along with efforts to fulfill today's short-term goals, simultaneous strategies are needed to build awareness with early physician recruits—to get ahead of the market curve. Also, we can no longer rely on single promotional sources to solicit candidates. Multiple vehicles with regular frequency are necessary to capture attention in a highly cluttered market space.

- Assigning internal leadership that reflects the professional talent level being sought. External firms can source for leads, but they can't contribute the organizational intuition, market knowledge, and strategic insights to deliver a well-positioned organization to candidates. Internal management is necessary—with the ability to guide and direct internal stakeholders through practice opportunity development, target identification, differentiated market messaging, and navigating diverse parties and interests through the recruitment process. Management attention also needs to be consistent to be effective—not in and out when the urgency arises.

- Measuring the effectiveness of the investment. With tracking and measurement tools in place, the organization builds internal history of what worked and what didn't. Recruitment efforts can then be refined and improved over time.

Just as efforts to improve quality, technology, and cost reduction require a defined plan with leadership guidance, today's competitive physician recruitment environment requires the same. That leadership investment prompts all stakeholders—including the organization's own medical staff—to recognize that physician recruitment is a serious strategic priority and is necessary to effectively compete in today's marketplace.

Physician retention

It's been estimated that the costs for one physician search fall in the range of $20,000 to $40,000, depending on the specialty, region of the country, and methods used. But that's just the start—organizations and/or practices can easily spend $100,000 by the time they consider all the expenses associated with the interviews and start up. Additional costs for income guarantees or practice set up are on top of that—it's expensive. Yet it drives patient care and, therefore, revenue. According to a Merritt Hawkins study, a doctor is worth about $1.54 million per year, ranging from pediatrics at $690,000 to more than $3 million for cardiovascular surgery. We need to recruit physicians, and it is an expensive undertaking, so what is in place to retain them?

Most of the time, losing a physician is rough. If the community was involved in the hiring effort, there is a personal sense of loss. The same holds true for the recruiter and the practice partners. A survey from national recruiting firm, Cejka Search, shows that more than half (54%) of physicians who leave their medical groups do so within the first five years. Everyone feels bad and replays their role and steps that could have been taken in hindsight. Retention also impacts care delivery, as often there is an added burden for other partners to pick up the patient load until a new physician is found. Likely, those who responded at a 3 or below in this survey had colleagues or partners that were not retained.

According to the Cejka survey, practice issues cause physicians to leave approximately 30% of the time, and compensation causes separation approximately 20% of the time. Other factors contributing to the issue of voluntary resignation for physicians include location (13%), spouse's career (10%), and the pressure of clinical practice (10%).

Again, senior executives do not need to be personally accountable, but they do need to set the example to ensure that the team members are trained, the team members have resources, and there are built-in accountabilities. If there are no repercussions for failing to implement retention strategies, good intentions fall by the wayside. Although there are whole books are written on retention, the following are some aspects where communication is key:

- Be picky; make sure that you hire for retention. If they do not seem like a fit, they probably are not. This is tough especially if you have had a position open for a period of time, but it is pain now or pain later.

- Clarify roles at the front end. This includes discussions with practice partners to detail how they will support the new physician.

- Discuss support that the organization will provide to assist with practice building. Call out your organization's role, and theirs.

- Commit to a formal on-boarding process. Consider a three-year plan, with special emphasis on year one. Call out areas that need mastery for the new doctor to feel success.

    - Personal connections are part of good on-boarding. Regular meetings that go beyond asking, "How's it going?" are critical.

    - Feedback and mentoring are valued by new physicians.

    - Acclimating to the community, the medical staff, and the family's move are important.

- The final area that is very much under the leader's control is practice experience at the facility. Make certain that promises made are kept, that there is respect for new practice patterns, and that the hospital environment is welcoming.

With impending physician shortages, it is likely that retention will become more important. As leaders, make sure that your team has a plan in place to acclimate the new doctors. Make certain that the doctor understands and buys into the plan, so that it is done with them rather than for them. And make certain that when a physician decides to leave, there is thorough review and steps are taken so mistakes are not repeated.

Obligations for retention extend deeply into the responsiveness of the medical staff. It is rare that a doctor could feel fulfilled in any type of practice setting without a connection to the other staff members. Sometimes physicians recognize the value of this—and clearly understand the approach. At other times, not so much! When in doubt, find ways to have your recruiter, physician relations rep, or on-boarding specialist spend the time to make certain that the medical staff and practice are welcoming and supportive.

Understand First

Many of the areas of this survey question boil down to the need to understand your physicians at a business level. Messages about "us" work better when we understand their point of view. Learn how practices function, how they engage with their patients, how staffing has changed, the business challenges of managing practice, and the impact of government changes on their specialty. Once you do this, then consider the business relationship that the physician has with your organization. Really step back and assess how the relationship works, and how it could be better for *both* parties. If you don't do this, it does not matter that you are a really nice person or that you take good care of your nursing staff.

Personal relationship building adds value after there is business credibility in place. When it is time to build a personal relationship, refuse to consider that all physicians are the same. All physicians have their own reason for choosing medicine, their own challenges in practice building and managing dollars, and their own personalities and approaches to dealing with patients. A leader who communicates well with the medical staff will explore each facet and then customize how the doctor receives communication. And, if you think it is too much work, consider how much effort is currently wasted because communication is about talking *at* someone.

Aligning for the Future

The responses to this survey question do more than simply share perceptions about how competitive the organization is in the eyes of the doctor. The results give us a glimpse into their perception of "what counts." This survey question was designed to discern the here and now, whereas the next chapter more fully addresses the views of alignment and the future.

A good leader knows that change requires physician buy-in and more often than not, buy-in to something tangible—like great quality, a strong medical staff, or trust in the patient care experience. Through communication, there is the opportunity to engage physicians in these strategies. Messages must be designed to be relevant to the needs of the doctor first and to their patients, rather than being about value for the organization.

Technology is discussed in terms of physician efficiency and the ability of existing specialists to do a procedure that was previously referred out. Patient care experience is tracked to show less repeat admissions—fewer pages for the physicians on call. You get the picture.

Good leaders very much appreciate involved and engaged doctors. Some do a marvelous job of involving them through conversations that are personally meaningful. Those who continue to talk about the organization without making the link find it more challenging to have physicians willing to engage in conversations about change.

Summary

Most hospital–leader communication patterns are the product of years of the same methods and sensitivity on both sides. Leaders are focused on the long-term viability of the organization, whereas many physicians are looking to the immediate needs for effective care delivery.

We've all heard the phrase, "Actions speak louder than words." Mother was right again. It's about that obligation to act on our promises. When that does not happen, it creates a cloud of skepticism.

If there is interest in garnering physicians' opinions, then the expectation is that they would be asked and listened to, and that their input would influence the action. If it can't happen that way, they would at minimum expect to know this. It's not just leadership and doctors—it is lots of individuals in many roles. It is just in this role that the leadership and operations teams want a little win to demonstrate their willingness to involve physicians. To begin or reinvent this process, find a way to ask a question in an area where you know you can be responsive. And don't forget—this is about gaining momentum, interest, and trust. Not easy; just necessary.

Many leaders are interested in more physician involvement. It makes sense as organizations collaborate on quality, safety, technology, and measures of success.

The ability to start with the business relationship and then leverage their personal needs is what allows us to earn a relationship that is beyond need fulfillment, beyond quenching the immediate thirst. This is where we begin to work in collaboration to provide value for the physician beyond the basic 8:00 a.m. block time in the operating room. Make a checklist of some ways you can add additional value. It may not be that every physician has a long list, but there are some that absolutely merit this activity. And sometimes it's just showing the willingness to make a list that makes the difference.

3

ACOs, PHOs: Industry Change and Physicians' Priorities in the Relationship

Contributing writer: Michael Barber, MD, with Barlow/McCarthy.

It is clear that physicians absolutely want to be involved in the development and implementation of an accountable care organization (ACO), including the policies, criteria, and measurement (see Figure 3.1). And the most important aspect of this hospital–physician relationship is the degree of control the physicians will have, according to 78% of the survey respondents. It is clear that organizations will do well to actively involve the physicians from the onset as this message is about doing with vs. having the process done and told to them.

On a personal level, the doctors rated physician performance and the distribution of shared savings and/or quality incentives as important, with scores of 43% and 41%, respectively.

Physicians want to hear early and often about their role in creating a collaborative model for accountable care.

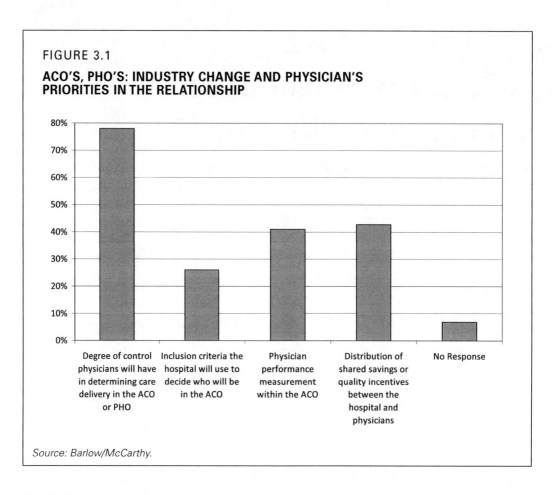

FIGURE 3.1

ACO'S, PHO'S: INDUSTRY CHANGE AND PHYSICIAN'S PRIORITIES IN THE RELATIONSHIP

Source: Barlow/McCarthy.

ACO Aware

What is surprising to me about this data is that just 6.9% of physicians failed to respond to this question. In a recent Reuters survey of nearly 3,000 physicians in September 2010, 45% of physicians indicated that they did not know what an ACO was much less had an opinion of what role they might play in an ACO.

The Complete Guide to Physician Relationships

Our response rate to this question may well represent selection bias of who completed the survey and indicate that these physicians are more aware and actively involved in shaping care in their communities today. As we move forward, there is a need for the healthcare system and hospital leaders not only to educate themselves and their hospital boards about the evolving ACO models and regulations but also to make this a joint learning process with their medical staff.

Forming joint physician/hospital exploratory committees, sending out ACO briefs, and presenting at departmental and medical staff meetings can all be effective ways to get the word out on the latest ACO news. It is very important to make sure that the hospital's direction in formation of ACO is communicated.

The Patient Protection and Affordable Care Act passed in 2010 is very broad in terms of how physicians and/or hospitals might go about organizing an ACO. Hospital/physician ACOs are likely to take many different forms. Let's dig into the data to see what aspects of hospital-based ACOs physicians are concerned about.

Degree of control in care delivery

Seventy-eight percent of respondents indicated that this topic is of overwhelming importance and concern to physicians. Physician autonomy in determining care delivery is a core value of physicians and is fiercely defended. Many states have corporate-practice-of-medicine statues that prohibit anyone other than an individual physician from making clinical decisions. This is a long standing and defended role.

*Physicians are concerned that the hospital ACO will become
the new overseer in the new hospital ACO relationship.*

In the *HealthLeaders Media 2010 Intelligence Unit Report* "Physician Alignment
in an Era of Change," 42% of hospital leaders indicated that ACO formation
would strain their relationship with physicians. Although there may be other
factors of ACO formation that strain hospital–physician relationships, the high
degree of importance to our survey respondents would indicate that physician
control of clinical care delivery will be front and center in physicians' minds when
approached about participating in an ACO.

Learning from the past

Some physicians are quick to point out the experience of the 1990s "mangled
care" debate, where care and costs were managed by having physicians jump
through hoops and hurdles when providing care. Primary care physicians (PCP)
referral requirements and onerous, time-consuming preauthorization procedures
combined with difficult "black box" claims adjudication systems drove physicians
and their patients crazy at times.

A lot has been learned since the 1990s about how to get better outcomes without
resorting to ineffectual and objectionable managed care techniques. New approaches can be considered based on organizational culture and market dynamics. Some
of these include the following:

* Transition of care management

* Improved patient self-management

- Patient-centered medical home

- Predictive modeling

- Just-in-time clinical interventions

In a recent physician meeting on a hospital's ACO strategy, one physician proclaimed, "The only answer is rationing." Answers like that or references to going back to 1990s managed care are a call for leaders to define the difference. Many integrated health systems and medical home practices are effectively improving care and lowering costs in a new model.

Involved discussions

A good approach is for health systems leaders to conduct exploratory educational sessions with their physician leaders. When possible, have the process led by a community physician. Such explorations can be done through literature searches, attending ACO conferences together, or working with an outside consultant who has implemented clinical intervention systems.

Shared Savings and Quality Incentives

What may surprise some is that shared savings and quality incentives did not rank first with nearly 43% of respondents raising this issue, but it is certainly a topic leaders are aware of as they approach physicians about participating in their ACO. It seems safe to assume that in markets where hospitals and physicians compete on many fronts—such as ambulatory surgery centers, imaging centers, and

INSIDER'S VIEW

WALK BEFORE RUNNING

Rick Tyler, MD, vice president medical affairs/CMO at CHRISTUS Health's southeast Texas region, shares his view on securing physician support.

"We have to walk before we can run. Before skeptical physicians will embrace any broad-scale shared financial risk associated with ACOs, they will need to feel comfortable with hospitals and physicians working collaboratively on smaller scale projects, and will need to see real success in improving quality and reducing costs."

These local market-driven opportunities would include service-line gainsharing ventures, varying degrees of comanagement arrangements, and clinical integration models involving smaller, defined populations, Tyler explains, adding that dyad management approaches with hospital executive and community physician leader working side-by-side have been shown to be the best approach in fostering mutually beneficial physician–hospital alignment and meaningful clinical integration. "Our initial approach has been to evaluate the local market, provide education to all stakeholders, and work from a standpoint of shared benefit—for hospital, physician, patient, and the healthcare system. We have also found The Advisory Board Company helpful in educating and facilitating discussions with community physicians. Physicians seem to be more responsive to an unbiased source of information."

laboratories—the economics of the relationship may need definition before the physicians are willing to consider participation.

With the requirement for hospitals and physicians in ACOs to be members of a separate joint organization, both parties will be positioning themselves to have control over the financial decisions to be made in how shared savings and potentially risk payments will be distributed. Complicating this from the physician's perspective, they are very concerned about how the physician portion of any savings will be distributed among the different medical specialties, especially because most believe that Medicare physician reimbursement will remain the same at best and may well be reduced in the near future.

Framing an approach

At present, there are no really good examples in healthcare that show us an ACO. Today's prepaid medical groups, like Kaiser Permanente, might be considered; however, those organizations operate almost entirely under a value-based reimbursement model and will not have to navigate the difficult waters of being reimbursed in the fee-for-service model that most hospitals and physicians are so familiar with and, at the same time, have a small portion of their reimbursement be value-based. With no good models to emulate, hospital and physician leaders alike need to look outside of healthcare to come up with their solution for how to divide the pie.

Volume-based vs. value-based

Healthcare is different from many other industries in that our economics have been volume-based and not value-based in any respect. Almost all other unregulated services and products are priced and sold on perceived or real demonstrated value. For instance, we purchase cars on multiple value dimensions—appearance, durability, mileage, and status symbol. No car manufacturer produces the value statements all on their own; rather, they buy products and services that go into creating a car from a variety of vendors and manufacturers. Manufacturers pay vendors (distribute a portion of the purchase price) based on the value the supplier adds to the finished product. Some of the value is created by the product they produce—zinc-coated steel for bodies that eliminate corrosion, for example—whereas other value is created by services provided, such as advertising and marketing, planning, and implementation, and yet other value is created by systems such as robotic assembly lines that improve quality and consistency.

Granted, healthcare is not the same as building and selling automobiles. Automobile sales and use is quite different from healthcare, but determining value and rewarding the producer based on the value added has a number of parallels in how you approach this issue.

For instance, the PCP who has high levels of patient adherence to antihypertensive and lipid management drugs in some cases may bring greater value to a system of care by reducing the number of patients having heart attacks and strokes than the cardiologist who performs life saving angioplasty on patients who, even in spite of the best care, have an acute cardiovascular event. However, if that PCP were able to produce increased adherence using a disease registry provided by the hospital and health coaches employed by the hospital, the hospital would have created value for the physician and should claim a portion of the value that was a result of that physician's patient treatment.

The proposed ACO regulations do provide two options for participating in the shared savings program. The one-sided option means that the ACO providers would be paid fee-for-service Medicare rates and only have an upside financial opportunity. The two-sided option and has upside and downside risks with the upside opportunity being larger than in the one-sided option. The two-sided option does have equity requirements to assure CMS that organizations can financially take the risk. It seems likely that many hospital and physician organizations will choose the one-sided option to ease concerns about how the parties will split the shared savings, because the payout will probably be small at the beginning stages and organizations won't have to deal with difficult issues, such as how they will share the potential losses between the hospital and physicians in the two-sided option. Having the opportunity to focus on care delivery redesign rather than money distribution, will be important to many ACOs in their formative years.

Is this a simple fact-based issue? No, of course not. But by using some of the analytic tools and systems used in other industries, hospitals and physicians can begin the dialogue on how they will resolve this difficult issue.

- Healthcare leaders will do well to paint a picture of learning, with choices to be made

- Communication will need to spell out how little we know about ACOs and shared savings reimbursement

- Conversation will be shaped to frame collaboration as new lessons surface about how physicians and hospitals will be rewarded in this newly emerging value-based reimbursement models today

- Exploring how other industries have determined value, hospitals and physicians can have a dialogue and answer the question of how they will make these critical decisions even though they cannot specifically answer "What dollars are in it for me?"

Joint exploration, education, and communication of this issue with physicians are the strategies with which healthcare systems are most likely to find the answers for their medical communities.

Physician Performance Measurement

The importance of this issue in physicians' minds was barely edged out by their concerns about the economics of ACOs, with 41% of respondents indicating that this is an important topic. This is not a new issue. Physicians have resisted measurement and comparison to their peers and to national standards for years. Insurance companies, managed care companies, and HMOs have attempted to change physician behavior by measuring various elements of care, comparing them to peers, and tying them to financial incentives with little success. The physician complaints are consistent: "My patients are sicker," "these results are from a claims analysis black box and are not reflective of my care and outcomes," and "this is about saving money, not improving care."

There is some truth to these complaints, but even if these observations are not accurate, physicians in ACOs will resist similar measurement systems coming from hospitals just as they have from insurance companies. Although it is tempting to use some of the readily available claims analysis tools to measure physician performance, healthcare leaders should consider evaluating physician behaviors that are linked to creating the high value outcomes that ACOs will need to produce to be successful.

Care coordination

Current research clearly demonstrates that improving care coordination, transitions of care from the acute hospital, and communication between providers will improve clinical outcomes. Each of these requires measurable behaviors from physicians for success.

Transition planning: In transitioning a patient from the acute care hospital to home or post acute care, the physician coordinates with the transition care team and documents the post hospital plan of care. This is communicated to the patient and/or caregivers. With care coordination, the obligation to complete timely discharge summaries and a structured transition plan can reduce the likelihood that the patient will be readmitted unnecessarily or suffer avoidable harm once they leave the hospital.

Physician to physician communication: Another example of a behavior that improves the efficiency and outcomes of care is getting physicians to communicate with one another more effectively. Communication between physicians often breaks down in both directions, and the consequences can lead to redundant testing as well as poorly implemented treatment plans for patients.

If an organization is to use physician performance measurement and management to improve care, they need to measure and manage two things:

1.   Physician participation in key elements of care systems designed to ensure better outcomes. An example would be transitions of care.

2. Physician adherence to evidenced-based care. An example here is beta-blocker use after myocardial infarction.

These behaviors and actions can be indisputably measured and managed far better than many of the claims-based measures that have been used in the past. As in the other areas of importance to physicians, physician participation in creating the measures is critical, as is having physician leaders create the expectation that their peers achieve high performance on the measures. As a leader, is there an opportunity to support physician leaders to initiate these discussions?

ANSWERING THE QUESTION

There is nothing easy about all of this for today's leaders. Keeping the physicians informed and engaged is what they want. Yet, there is recognition that the hospital will need to make some choices. Beyond conversations, data and past patterns will come into play. Some of this feels almost reminiscent of getting selected for a sand lot baseball team. Now that the proposed ACO regulations were released on March 31, 2011, some elements have greater definition, but many hospital-physician issues are still waiting to be solved. Some leaders have opted to lay out the potential elements and then potential action. Visual tools to show options always work well as an approach with physicians.

Inclusion criteria the hospital will use

Although this aspect of the hospital–physician relationship received the fewest votes as being important, it still was selected by 26% of the physicians. Of those indicating that inclusion criteria were important, about half were specialists and half PCPs. The following are some of those up in the air issues:

The Complete Guide to Physician Relationships

- The proposed Medicare ACO regulations do specify that patients will be virtually enrolled based on their previous patterns care and which primary care physicians provide most of their primary care services. ACOs will be given lists of potential Medicare beneficiaries that are based on previous years of Medicare claims, but the actual calculation of shared savings will be based on which patients are virtually enrolled for measurement year. To make the process even more complicated, the ACO regulations specify that the ACO cannot restrict or present barriers to any enrolled person's choice or location of services. This means that patients can go to any physician or choose any hospital at any time. It appears that hospitals will want to include as many PCPs in their ACO as possible since patient enrollment will be determined by the PCP that a Medicare patient is seeing and PCPs can only participate in one ACO.

- This would seem to indicate that hospitals will use the size of a PCP's Medicare patient panel as initial screening criteria in deciding who should be in their panel.

- A second screen should be patient satisfaction scores for Medicare patients in a PCP's practice because there is high correlation between satisfaction scores, patient loyalty, and adherence to physician recommendations—all necessary to keep patients voluntarily within the health system.

- Hospitals will want to consider including primary care practices that demonstrate that they can work in coordinate care systems and be effective in primary and secondary preventive care.

IN THE MEANTIME

As the stage is being set for new models of care delivery and the dynamics continue to percolate, hospital strategists and physician relations specialists can be instrumental in conditioning the physician–hospital relationship for what's potentially to come. Consider the following activities today:

- Keep your brand strong to gain credibility with the physician network; they want to be aligned with a partner with a strong brand

- Market to your physicians; consider them a key audience, and position your clinical differentiators using messages and tools that make an impact

- Actively communicate with them, and ask for their opinions and input; keep them informed

- Support their practice development where you can; demonstrate your interest in helping them to succeed

- Build collaboration with physicians; involve them in organizational decision-making; recruit physician champions for operational and clinical initiatives

- Utilize your physician relations staff to help identify needs and expectations and then to engage C-suite executives with key targets, as appropriate

- Connect with new physicians to the market; welcome them and get them engaged with your medical staff and facility quickly

- Those with data or experience from medical homes may well consider a physician's willingness or progress toward patient-centered medical home one of their inclusion considerations.

- One of the thornier issues hospitals will have to contend with is who is a PCP, especially with medical specialists and subspecialists who, for some patients, act as PCPs.

- With specialists having the ability to be in multiple ACOs, they will want to be in as many ACOs as possible. In today's world, hospitals try to woo specialists to perform as much of their work in their facilities as possible. However, under value-based reimbursement, hospitals will want specialists who will work with PCPs and hospital care coordinators to prevent unnecessary admissions to the acute care setting. This will be a big shift for hospitals to look for and will reward cooperation and collaboration over volume admitters.

Summary

Although you could debate whether ACOs or physician-hospital organizations (PHO) will reshape how healthcare is delivered in many of our communities, it is hard to argue with their intended goal of getting physicians and hospitals to work more closely together to produce better patient outcomes. Faced with an aging population and diminishing financial resources, it seems logical for hospitals and physicians to work toward improving the efficiency and quality of care together by following these principles:

1. Joint exploration and learning of ACOs and other collaborative care delivery models

2. Building of physician leadership capabilities so that physicians can responsibly assume control of that which is most important to them: how care is delivered

3. Develop a value-based methodology of shared financial decision-making

4. Measure and manage physician behaviors that are consistent with and/or support coordinated care

5. Develop physician behavior based criteria for inclusion

Following these principles will not be easy for hospitals or physicians but can help redefine the hospital–physician relationship and position both to be successful in meeting the demands of the future.

What Do Physicians Want to Hear From Their Peers?

"Two men in a burning house must not stop to argue."
–African Proverb

One would think that with all of the years spent in medical school and residency, physicians would have ample time working with each other to establish solid communication skills. In reality, however, good communication gets limited attention. Much about the referral process and messages to facilitate referral communication are learned by watching the patterns of others. Sometimes that is marvelous, but not always. When the physician is in training, the focus is on treating patients and learning. Little thought is given to earning referrals and understanding how and where they originate. Frankly, some physicians can go through their entire training—and often very successful careers—without having to consider the referral chain. For others, practice building is a daily reality. In specialty areas, the patients often see a primary care physician (PCP) who offers referral recommendations. Today, most specialists benefit from having good relationships with their colleagues—besides enhancing the care experience and patient outcomes, it can also enhance referrals.

It does not take much effort to appreciate the challenges surrounding communication for physicians, with their patients, staff, and individuals they work with in facilities. A word search of "communication" in the *Archives of Internal Medicine* sourced 4,552 articles with communication in the title. Everyone wants something from physicians—and their physician colleagues are no different.

This section is about referral communication expectations from one doctor to another. We also wanted to explore how connected physicians were to their key referral sources. Do they refer to those they know? Although the content is written for doctors, I recognize that many readers will be supporting the relationships. If your role is as a hospital employee, you'll hopefully find suggestions to nurture relationships from the sidelines. If you lead an employed group, the goal is to have discussions about referral relationships and approach *before* you hire a new physician. If you are in private practice, there is opportunity to define your group based on consistent and thoughtful communication.

LEGAL IMPLICATIONS

Whenever we talk about referral relationships, there is the trepidation of making sure all referral relationships are legal. The approach of connecting with other doctors, providing education, and sharing expertise is all legal. Actually, it is the right thing to do because the referring physician should be informed about service provided, the approach used, and the philosophy of the physician or team providing the service.

What is *not* legal are referral fees or payments to the doctor in exchange for a referral, commonly known as kickbacks. Federal law prohibits this, and many states also have laws to address this. Keep your focus on communication and everyone stays away from the ghastly orange jumpsuits.

Who Gets Picked?

The top three factors to determine who gets referrals are expertise, personal communication, and patient experience. Physicians ranked clinical expertise/quality as the No. 1 criterion they use when selecting specialists for their patients, with almost 90% selecting that variable (see Figure 4.1). This result is no surprise, but some may be surprised that it did not receive 100% of the vote, since they could select multiple criteria.

Referring physicians ranked communication second at 83%. About two-thirds of the physicians in this survey cited the importance of the patient's perception of their care experience. I wonder whether they are asking or if patients are simply volunteering this information. Right behind patient experience is ease of access for the patient at just under 60%. Location, travel, and the needs of the patient are coming into play more than we believed, historically.

Appointment access was important for 57% of physician respondents. That percentage makes it important, but perhaps it is surprising that physicians called out four other criteria more frequently.

Although physician promotion often highlights background training and experience, these were cited less often. The bottom score for physicians when they consider a specialist is their hospital affiliation. If you are a part of the hospital, you may want to evaluate whether this is good, bad, or neutral.

Note: These results include referrals both from PCPs to specialists and from specialists to other specialists.

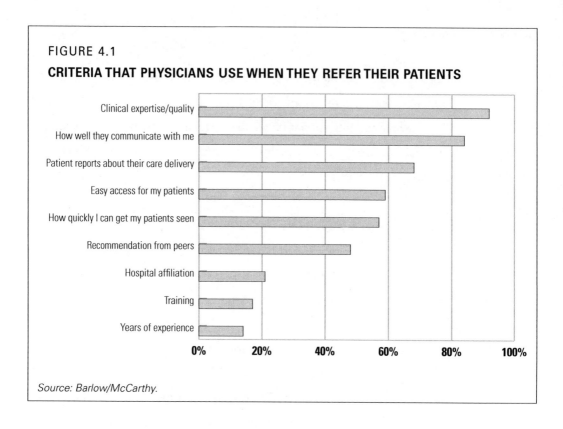

FIGURE 4.1

CRITERIA THAT PHYSICIANS USE WHEN THEY REFER THEIR PATIENTS

Source: Barlow/McCarthy.

Demonstrating Quality in a Peer-to-Peer Setting

The survey findings raise the interesting question, "How are referring physicians judging quality?" We understand that they expect clinical solutions for their patients (e.g., returning with the right diagnosis and treatment). But there is likely more to this. It is certainly a question that could and should be asked in the local market. A specialist should have a sense of the deciding factors that their referral sources use; for instance, do they refer all their patients to one doctor/group? Do they define referrals based on specialization? Do they switch up and, if so, what criteria do they

The Complete Guide to Physician Relationships

use? If you are uncertain how you were selected, it is okay to ask. It is also okay to learn about parameters and criteria. If you ask, then be prepared to respond with what they want. And when you ask, make certain that you give some choices or options so the question is comfortable and does not put them on the spot.

As a specialist, demonstrating quality as a part of education about services and techniques makes sense. It can't be braggadocios or it will backfire. But, if physicians currently refer to you and believe you have quality, reinforce it. If they are using another provider, your strong quality outcomes can differentiate you. This can be in personal meetings, as a part of educational meetings (e.g., continuing medical education, grand rounds, tumor board) or in similar meetings.

Some patients will ask about outcomes. Whatever data is shared with the patient or family should also be given to the referring physician. It need not be formal; include it in your "thank you for referring this patient" note after the visit. But make certain that the data you share is current, relevant, and accurate.

Encourage discussions with referring physicians about their perceptions of quality to understand how they are looking the topic today and how you may enlighten them regarding quality from within your specialty.

Nobody refers to bad quality doctors

No doctor sits in the exam room and says, "I think today I will refer Jane Doe to a doctor who has marginal quality." It is important to connect with this. Before any provider makes a referral, they have justified the quality. They may know that Dr. Adams has fellowship training in the field but believe that Dr. Fine has done that procedure for years. They may know that Dr. Smith is crabby but is the best clinically.

Quality can't just be talked about; it needs to be proven. The best communications approach is to talk about how you define quality and then show you meet that definition through data. It's not necessary to have comparative data from competitors. National benchmarks are nice, but the most important point is to have your data and to share the implications.

Consistent Communication

Eighty-three percent of physicians indicated that how they personally are communicated with by the specialist is a key criterion for referrals. Referring physicians expect communication about the patients they refer. That feels fair, doesn't it? Yet there are some significant challenges.

Linked electronic medical records (EMR) have done a great deal to streamline this process, and when all physicians are part of the EMR, it works great. But not everyone is part of the EMR. In addition, knowing the challenges that many organizations face in tracking primary care referral data, this number is frightening. The assumption is that practices are capturing referring physician names rather than relying on the hospital organization's record. It's a chronic challenge: Communication can't take place if there is no record of who referred the patient. With or without the EMR, for organizations or individual doctors, passing referral information off and believing it is not a priority is the wrong thing to do.

INSIDER'S VIEW

COMBATING OLD MYTHS

"These survey findings gave me some new insights to some very old myths," says Phillip M. Kibort, MD, MBA, vice president medical affairs and chief medical officer at Children's Hospitals and Clinics of Minnesota. "We used to think that docs wanted, in order, availability, affability, and then ability. This survey indicates that statement has been turned 180 degrees. Clinical expertise and communication reigns supreme. It will be helpful for me."

Everyone can ask

It is not just one person's job to capture the name of the referring physician. If the admitting clerk or office staff does not fill in the blank, then the nurse can ask. And if the doctor interviews the patient and there is no note of the referring physician, he or she can ask, too. Even when a patient self-refers for specialty care, ask if it's okay to keep their personal physician in the loop.

A simple practice that has shored up this area for some organizations is to acknowledge that many patients don't relate to the term PCP. Ask, "Who do you see for colds and flu?" Learn when they last saw them, and take the time to make certain it is captured in their record.

Patients talk

Patients talk, and the talk is about everything. At yoga class today, one of the attendees offered both referral advise and treatment recommendations for another yogi. Likely, the knowledge was misguided, but it was assertive and believable.

Beyond sharing with friends and colleagues, patients are quick to share their experiences with the physician who referred them for additional care. Ask yourself, "How can you better leverage this communication?"

The survey affirms that physicians listen to what their patients say about their referral experience. Physicians who are interested in growing a practice through referrals from other specialists can benefit from a proactive plan to enhance the chances of the right message flowing back to the initial referrer.

Take an extra five minutes at discharge to remind patients of their procedure, and ask them on a scale of one to five how they rate their care, their overall experience, and you personally. Suggest that when they see their doctor, they greet him or her on your behalf and tell them the type of note he or she will receive.

Check on paperwork, and remind patients that they have the right to ask about it, too. If the patient is being discharged from the hospital and the discharge instructions are not yet in place when final rounds are complete, then tell the patient that an envelope should accompany them (if it is a patient that will need to be seen again soon).

When you have a chance to speak with your referring doctors, ask about the feedback they get from patients. And of course, never say to a patient anything that you do not want repeated about a referring physician!

Making It Easy for Patients

The physician's perception of what's easy for their patients is influenced by what they have learned from other patients and their own perceptions. Some of the most common considerations are location, proximity to other healthcare services, and providers and family needs.

Realtors have long ascribed to the adage: location, location, location. The location of the practice will impact referral patterns in a positive or negative way. Evaluate both. If distance is an issue, the practice will need to look at the geographic market that they wish to reach and make some business decisions. Does a satellite office make sense? Do we work harder in our immediate area? Although people will drive and they will pass other clinics to get to a specialist, it's always harder and requires more clinical specialization. It also requires more work for the personal physician—are you worth it?

Academic medical centers have been challenged with location and the drive in to the city, some with parking, and many with sheer size and complexity of the campus. Spend time with referral coordinators, and offer tools and services to enhance the ease for patients if it is a challenge you face.

Defining access

For many practices and busy specialists, the topic of appointment access is exhausting and frustrating—they will tell you everyone wants to be seen immediately for everything. Physician relations staff will be quick to tell which specialties are a problem. Based on this research, is it a problem that impacts referrals? Yes or no, doing it better is always the goal.

At the heart of physician access, perhaps there is a bit of ego. For the primary care referral source there is a desire to show the patient that they are able to quickly respond on their behalf. For the specialist, the fact that patients are backed up is a nod to their expertise and short-term security for their stream of income. For both parties, it often comes down to communication.

SPECIALISTS GO DIRECT TO PATIENTS

In most markets there are specialty groups that have opted to go direct to consumers with their services and immediate access. Radio ads that offer immediate orthopedic care for sports injuries are a good example. You need to determine what the impact is on practice growth and on referral relations.

Involved decisions about time frame

Some patients wait better than others—they are wired to be more patient and less anxious. Some diagnoses are easier to sit on than others, and some referring physicians are just more anxious about their referrals than others. If your practice relies on referrals, it will be important to have staff trained to understand these differences. It can help to script language that staff can consistently use when discussing wait times both with patients and referring physicians.

Many busy practices have found ways to work around the perception of long waits for an appointment when a doctor refers to another doctor. Sometimes it is as easy as a five-minute physician-to-physician phone call. Sometimes it is a visit with another doctor or allied care professional, plus a greeting and action plan conversation with the selected specialist. Sometimes it is a nurse in the practice calling the patient to talk through plans and approach.

The starting point is to ask the referring physician when he or she believes the patient should be seen. A little shared control of the power goes a long way.

Track the number of physician calls for appointments and the access issues at a practice level. Make certain to monitor how long the waits are and set a red flag time for communication with everyone. For example, if the practice wait time for a new patient is longer than seven days, the practice manager and physicians will be notified. Talking to each other in the practice is essential if external communication is to be enhanced.

Some physicians just will not put up with chronic long waits, so business will decline. If you don't want that, then trend and respond with recruitment, a modification to patient flow and efficiencies in the office, a change of venue, or the size of the referral base.

Tangled Twine of Priorities

If you have access issues and no proactive plan, then the physician who witnessed the wait will tell their peers. In the same way, communication issues will be packaged as an issue of quality. The referral source will say, "I cannot provide quality care without knowing what happened at ACME General."

Word of mouth is a strong tool within the physician rank and file. Those physicians who want to enhance their relationships with their peers would do well to think about how they are perceived on all these fronts.

Is there a role for training and experience?

From this study, it appears that training and experience are not strong difference makers when choosing the right specialist for a referral—perhaps they are assumed. The take-away is that if we have limited time to communicate with referring physicians, the time is better spent with clinical outcomes, approach to quality care, patient experience, and communication.

Should hospital affiliation count for more?

Hospital teams are probably more surprised by this low score than physicians. This has never been more evident than in the struggles that health systems face when working to earn referrals from those physicians they employ. With the push toward tighter affiliations, there will be an opportunity for marketers and leaders to work with physicians to more tightly define value. This could start with clinical outcomes that show a group of doctors at that hospital. It could call out the type of technology, patient satisfaction data, or patient experience tracking tool.

The impact here will likely occur with more comparative data and more intentional messaging at the quality, safety, and experiential level. For organizations that want that, it starts with data disseminated to the specialists and referring physicians. Given all of this, it is still important to remember that physicians refer to other physicians, not to the organization.

Maybe it's just the relationship

The insight provided by physicians gives us a good road map to build processes, tools, and messages to support the referral process between physicians. However, let's not forget that sometimes the referral relationship boils down to just that: the relationship.

For any of you who've tried to shift referral patterns or redirect referrals from a competitor's specialist to yours, you know that these relationships can be difficult to break, especially if it's a good relationship. This is because physicians get comfortable with what they know. Of course, clinical expertise/quality and timely communication is important, but sometimes that becomes secondary to the 20-year referral history between two physicians.

You need to understand and recognize these relationship nuances. Sometimes our best opportunity to support the referral process comes in the timing—perhaps when a physician becomes disgruntled with their current relationship, or a relationship ends because of an out-of-market move, or maybe your new specialist can provide something that is not being provided in the current relationship. This is where that list of specialty selection criteria comes in handy.

Summary

Kibort said it well: In today's environment, communication and quality make a difference in where referrals go. Some specialists are able to set their pace and their own patterns without consideration for the desires of the referring physician.

Many more recognize the role of the PCPs in their practice success. In both worlds, it seems the patient benefits from streamlined communication among the physician team. We all have egos, and we all want to do the right thing for patients. Communication about all aspects of care will enhance everyone's experience.

Referrals often come as a result of who you are, not just the clinical service you provide.

Do Physicians on the Medical Staff Know Each Other?

Physicians refer to who they know: A combined 90% of physicians say they are familiar with referral colleagues at their primary facility (see Figure 5.1).

As one may expect, according to our age analysis, only the youngest age group of physicians (less than 35 years) do not know the majority of physicians they refer to. Only 46% of this group know the physicians they refer to or the majority of the medical staff. For all other age groups, the percentage of physicians who know most of the medical staff jumps well above 50%, and even as high as 80% among some of the older age groups.

With the movement toward more hospitalist coverage and primary care physicians (PCP) spending limited time at the hospital, it may be surprising that just 9% of physicians indicated that they don't know many of the physicians. The specialty breakout suggests that specialists tend to know a majority of the medical staff at a slightly higher rate than PCPs, although the difference is small.

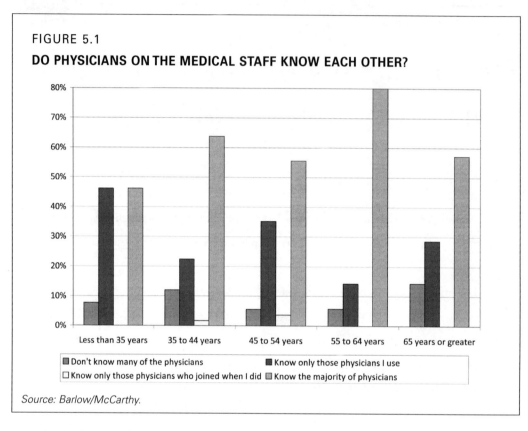

FIGURE 5.1

DO PHYSICIANS ON THE MEDICAL STAFF KNOW EACH OTHER?

Legend:
- Don't know many of the physicians
- Know only those physicians I use
- Know only those physicians who joined when I did
- Know the majority of physicians

Source: Barlow/McCarthy.

The findings and implications for this data are short and sweet. Knowing each other is important, and it matters whether they know you. There are many reasons why creating connections makes sense. The most obvious is that physicians are more inclined to think first of those doctors they know when they are making referral decisions.

Camaraderie and collegiality have long been hallmarks of the medical education system. Finding ways to allow this process to continue will create pathways for enhancing referral relationships, and it is the right thing to do. Everyone benefits.

The Complete Guide to Physician Relationships

Beyond shared discussions about procedures, a trusted relationship between physicians enhances dialogue about the patient condition, the right treatment regime, and the follow-up care.

Facilities can benefit from medical staff camaraderie as well because it can present a strategic opportunity to disseminate information. We have watched trusted, credible members of the medical staff reinforce positive messages or turned bad situations around for the hospital by serving as organizational ambassadors with other physicians. Physicians trust other physicians, especially when it comes to shaping their perspective and viewpoints about their partner facility.

Knowing and Referring

It is human nature to think first of those we know when someone is in need. If someone were to ask you for recommendations for getting your car serviced, the answer is probably a place you've used, even if you have heard there is a razzle-dazzle service center across town. Although clinical expertise plays a role in this equation, so does that desire to match a physician's style with the patient. Physicians will often say, "I always refer to John Doe when I have someone who needs more time and attention, or explanation." The ability to make these kinds of decisions is only possible if a referral relationship already exists.

Beyond working to make the right match, there is an assurance for the patient when their physicians can offer some personal detail about the specialist or group. It's a smart thing to do when there is opportunity.

For specialists who have a strong relationship with their referral source, the colleagues will often rely on them for phone consultation. Some doctors hate the thought of having other doctors call for opinions. Yet many doctors have built their referral base from this service. This is especially true when the expertise is in a niche area and the geographic draw makes a phone relationship the most efficient option.

Ease of Referral

The last chapter called out issues of access: how easy it was for the patients and how available the appointments were. The other element is simply top-of-mind awareness. As a physician communicates the need for a referral with a patient, it is easier to refer to "my colleague," and provide a name and detail. Sometimes the referral happens just because it is the person that the doctor knows best. As a recipient of referrals, you should have a sense of how many of your referrals come for that reason, and determine whether that is enough reason.

Payer

Relationships are rarely enough to overcome issues of payer incompatibility. Much has been written and studied in this regard. Suffice to say that it is important to understand the payer mix of those with whom you have a referral relationship. Staff should track the detail so there is solid understanding before contracts are due.

Be fed and feed

Beyond understanding payer issues, an inventory of relationships and referral sources is a good idea. For some practices, there may be a new relationship focus

The Complete Guide to Physician Relationships

if the data reveals that a large percentage of a certain type of referrals is coming from one practice. What do you know about that practice, their legacy, and their options for referral?

Physicians refer to those they know, but they also expect reciprocation. In other words, look for ways to feed those who feed you.

Market differences

Ann S. O'Malley, MD, MPH, and James D. Reschovsky, PhD, analyzed the 2008 Center for Studying Health System Change *Health Tracking Physician Survey* of 4,720 physicians for their January 2011 article in the *Archives of Internal Medicine*. Their analysis indicates that experience and the type of community in which a physician practices were major factors in how well doctors communicated. Physicians with 20 or more years of experience were more likely to report routinely sending and receiving information, as were physicians who worked in smaller, more rural communities.

Those who are in smaller communities get to know their medical neighbors. They rely on these relationships for their practice success. When it is more personal, then it is more important to close the loop and make sure that good communication is in place.

Welcome new physicians

With physician recruitment aggressively underway across the country, it is likely that new physicians are joining your medical staff as well. Take the opportunity to personally welcome your new colleagues. There's benefit to both PCPs and specialists—on one side, a new PCP can become a new referral source for the specialist and, on the other side, a new specialist may provide a unique clinical service that the PCP isn't already getting with currents members of the medical staff.

Elements That Impact Referral Decisions

Today, referring physicians certainly realize that they drive a large portion of referrals to specialists, to outpatient facilities, and to healthcare organizations. Although there are personal nuances about method and time frame, there are some certainties across the continuum.

Many physicians have heard or witnessed a story from a physician who referred a patient to a specialist only to have communication breakdown. For example, the physician runs into a family member at the local grocery store to learn that the patient died. You just can't make that up; it really happens. They don't all die, but procedures are done, specialists are consulted, and life-changing decisions are made without a note back to the personal referral source. By hearing examples with real patients attached and seeing the frustration and sadness in the eyes of the referring physician, the hope is that we find ways to avoid this.

No doctor ever intends this to be the case, so how does it happen? Likely everyone got busy, and there was a failure to track the referral source or get the note sent with changes. In the case of a death, perhaps the specialist assumed the hospital would make the call and that did not happen. It is not about casting blame; it is about understanding how gaps in communication can impact relationships. Embarrassment is just very hard on relationships. Personal experience tells me the best chance for re-earning the referral relationship is to have a personal connection and, of course, an acknowledgment.

Tangible and intangible influencers

Factors outside of the physician-to-physician referral relationship can impact referral decisions. Consider customer service at the clinic and/or hospital, if it's inpatient. In the practice setting, the physician may be disconnected from the practice experience. Long waits, lack of courtesy or support by staff, or challenges with accessing the practice may be enough for the patient to ask for another referral choice, or to find one on their own. Although these factors are often outside the control of the relationship we're talking about here, it's still something organizational leaders should consider.

The referrer has skin in the game too

A lot of the communication techniques recommended to this point have been about the obligation of the specialist who is working to earn referrals. No relationship will work when there is only one person interested in its success.

Strong referral relationships are built on mutual respect. For the specialist, this means receiving good workups and documentation when a patient is referred. The referring physician needs to take the time to package the chart. But some of the copied charts could fill a wheelbarrow, so take the time to highlight the reason for the referral, including current lab or other test results that support the decision.

There is sensitivity to ensuring that referrals are not given exclusively by payer, so one specialist gets only patients with less desirable, or no, insurance. Make sure to factor in the timing of referral too so that the patient is sent in time to be able to improve the clinical condition, rather than hanging on to the patient and only referring at the crisis point.

Some physicians aren't great referral partners, so decisions need to be made about that on both sides. Nobody wants to be taken advantage of. If your practice often refers out, take the time to examine how the process works and standardize some protocol. Consider who calls, what to ask for, the type of information that should be sent with the patient, and the patient's comprehension at the time of referral. For those with whom the referral relationship is strong, ask, "Is there additional information we should be sending that would help you?" Don't assume. Work to learn and accommodate to the needs of both parties; the patient will win, and so will both of the practices.

GETTING TO KNOW YOU

- There has to be value

- Make it easy: be available, be welcoming

- Fun is okay

- Personal and professional interests count

- Don't press

- Stay in touch; offer gentle reminders that you're still there

- Communicate, consistently

- Observe those you wish to meet interacting with others

A little social is okay

Many doctors will tell you that they hate the extra meetings and the social stuff—after a full day of work, many healthcare professionals just want their home, family, and a nice chair—not a piece of chicken and chit chat. Still, strong relationships at the local level benefit from some personal connectivity. We understand that physicians will feel more comfortable collaborating with or referring to those physicians that they connect with on a social level.

The hospital will offer some standard options of meetings, educational venues, and often a few social outings. If that does not work, consider personal connections with a select list. Or suggest other venues and other times to the hospital event planners. Determine a set amount of social time that will be devoted to practice development and networking. Stay consistent with it. Give it a chance to work by meeting new people each time. Follow up, and create a relationship. It really can happen with limited pain if you give it a chance.

One level deeper

Then there are physicians that are going to need some guidance in all of these elements. At a fundamental level, they understand the importance of the relationship but may just not know how to go about building and nurturing it. This is where the marketing team, physician relations team, and/or practice managers come in. These individuals may know best about the personalities and styles of the physicians to be able to effectively match them up with others. And physicians will appreciate ideas and suggestion for making the connections.

Summary

I asked Eric Engwall, managing partner at E.G. Insight, Inc., to weigh in on the topic of loyalty. Their company implements feedback processes that yield deeper understanding of the current health of critical business relationships. He shared that, "When it comes to referrals, true loyalty is more than just a matter of convenience or behavior borne out of habit. If there's no real connection between the referring party and the entity being referred, that relationship is vulnerable to simple changes in experience, routine, or environment. When a person makes a referral, whether for a physician or a restaurant, they put their own reputation on the line. Therefore, referral behavior is based on trust and confidence—confidence in the ability to provide good outcomes for the patient and trust that the overall patient experience will be positive. Without those emotional elements of trust and confidence, the first unsatisfactory experience may cause the next referral to go to someone or someplace else."

For the most part, doctors know each other. Although the survey did not detail the type of relationship and the methods for developing that relationship (e.g., phone, face-to-face), the results clearly indicate that the majority of physicians still feel that connection to others on the medical staff.

Those physicians who refer and those who want referrals will benefit from tending to the relationship, as all relationships do. The best way to do this is to understand what makes it work best for the other party and then work to achieve that goal.

6

Communication When a Referral Is Sent

Communication of some type regarding referred patients is crucial to physicians—especially primary care physicians (PCP), who are less likely to see their patients in the hospital due to the growing presence of hospitalists. It is critical for PCPs to receive discharge notification, as evidenced by Figure 6.1. In fact, 100% of PCPs want a full discharge summary that includes patient status and a medication report. PCPs also want to be notified when one of their patients is admitted to the hospital (78%) or seen by a specialist (66%).

Specialists also value and expect periodic updates on their patients, although the type of communication desired is somewhat different than what PCPs want. Receiving updates when the patient is seen by another physician is most important to specialists (72%), whereas just more than 50% want a full discharge summary. Many specialists want to be notified of major events or changes in patient status as well. Admission notices are less important because most patients are admitted at the request of the specialist.

For some physicians, access to an electronic medical record (EMR) alleviates some of the need for paperwork, and the ability to access the patient's full record

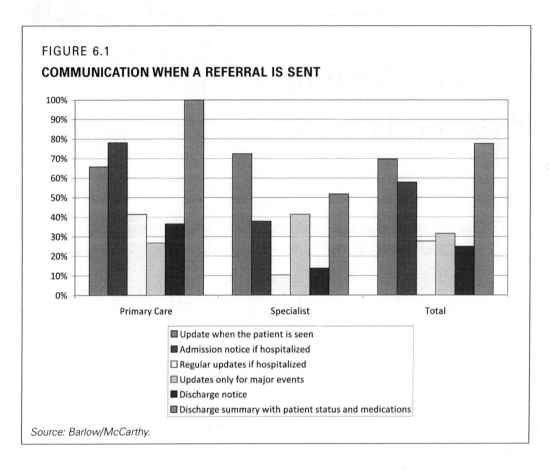

FIGURE 6.1

COMMUNICATION WHEN A REFERRAL IS SENT

Source: Barlow/McCarthy.

through a portal or shared system has certainly streamlined the process and enhanced communication.

An article in the *Archives of Internal Medicine* (January 10, 2011) shared survey results from 4,720 doctors that are worth noting as we explore referral communication. That study found significant variation between PCPs' and specialists' perceptions of the frequency in which they send and receive information on patients for referrals and consultations.

Although 69.3% of PCPs said they send specialists notification of a patient's history and the reason for the consultation all or most of the time, just 34.8% of specialists said they routinely receive such information, according to the study. Meanwhile, 80.6% of specialists say they send consultation results to the referring physician all or most of the time, but only 62.2% of PCPs say they ever receive that information.

That is a large discrepancy among a large number of physicians. The actual correspondence is probably somewhere in between, but this perception complicates matters and adds to the challenge of determining what we should do and what we need, and what others do and what they need.

Care Delivery Postdischarge

Being alerted when patients you refer are discharged from the hospital seems like a reasonable request. It also assumes that the specialist has records from the referring doctor, which eases the correspondence loop. For physicians who refer a large number of patients and who are not on an EMR, include a simple note that says, "Please e-mail or fax details of John Doe's treatment to Dr. Mary Smith, *msmith@acme.edu* or 111/222-3333." Practices that outline their expectations at the time of referral increase the likelihood of receiving the desired response.

It all boils down to notification for a quarter of the physicians surveyed. One could speculate that this is because they have access to the patient record through an EMR or they are one of a group of attending physicians that will have limited follow-up postdischarge.

When the physician is expected to provide follow-up care, then the details count. Assuming an EMR is not an option, discharge notes for hospitalized patients are usually prepared by the facility. Physicians are challenged—okay, frustrated—when this does not occur.

Every party owns responsibility for getting the discharge report sent to the physician. Organizations should have a protocol and defined steps in the process to give this communication consistency and reliability. You can assess this process to determine where the breakdown occurs and how often, with the following steps:

- Track calls into medical records, or if you capture this at the facility's call center, track it there too.

- Put the numbers to it. Show how many times in a month/quarter it is not managed as intended.

- Ask the physician relations representative to track the frequency of this complaint.

- Use the data to define whether it is a systemwide, department-specific, or even shift-specific error.

If it is a chronic complaint, then it is a systems issue, not a personnel issue. Consider it a quality/safety issue, and use your internal processes to fix it. What this data tells us is that failure to do so is a big deal. It reflects poorly on the institution, and perhaps more poorly on the discharging physician. Neither party wants to be in that position.

It all takes time

The lack of communication is rarely intentional. With the pace of clinical practice, the number of locations, and all of the messages being communicated from a variety of mediums, there is simply not enough time. Studies indicate that the average PCP spends between 10 and 18 minutes with their patients, and most have their schedules booked without breaks. Specialists are often serving multiple locations, and they will often rely on hospital staff to communicate with the referral source. Unless concerns are raised, PCPs and specialists alike assume that records are being sent and notes are accompanying the discharge. Office managers have full plates, too. But someone needs to track discharge communication to understand its frequency and impact. This is not just about doing it right because of the on-going desire to earn those referrals—there are patient care issues at play as well.

INSIDER'S VIEW

THE COMMUNICATION PROCESS SHOULD BE AUTOMATIC AND PERSONAL

There are examples of physicians doing this right in markets all over the country. Some have learned by example, some intuitively understand the benefits of great communication, and, for many, it's a combination of both factors. One Mayo-trained physician we work with—Aaron Altenburg, MD, with Idaho Orthopaedic & Sports Clinic in Pocatello, ID—is such a physician. Altenburg's desire to form good relationships with referring physicians materialized during his residency and fellowship. Although he is focused on developing his clinical and patient care skills, he instinctively knows that the relationship with referring physicians is important, too. So he actively watched how surgeons were communicating with other physicians and quickly recognized that for himself, as a busy surgeon, communication needed to be focused and implemented with intent. It didn't take him long to learn what worked and what didn't from the referring physicians' perspective.

INSIDER'S VIEW

THE COMMUNICATION PROCESS SHOULD BE AUTOMATIC AND PERSONAL (CONT.)

That knowledge, combined with his commitment to provide the best medical care possible, motivated Altenburg to pay close attention to his relationships with referring physicians. His objective is to make the communication process automatic and personal. To Altenburg, the simple act of a face-to-face introduction is vital. He hopes that he can help the physicians feel confident in sending patients to him once they have had a chance to meet him. That's how he develops the initial relationship.

To build on that relationship, he knows a big part of long-term success comes down to the all-important communication on referred patients. He takes a customized approach. In his practice, every physician is contacted in one way or another. On top of that, he factors variables such as the complexity of the case and his current relationship and expectations of the referring physician to determine whether additional layers of communication should be used. For example, he will often call the physician directly to discuss a particular case. Location of the referring physician is also an important factor he considers because of his sensitivity to the rural markets that surround his. Altenburg understands rural physicians prefer that one-to-one contact, so he accommodates them.

Beyond patient communication, Altenburg stays in regular contact with his physician network through educational programs and by simply being accessible should his consultative services be needed.

Is his strategy paying off? Yes, says Altenburg. He knows this because he and hospital staff hear it directly from the physicians. He has become a resource to them, getting consultation and referral calls directly even when he's not on call. He is building physician relationships in markets where there haven't been such relationships historically, and where he knows that fewer patients are being referred out of the local market. In the end, referring physicians show their appreciation by sending Altenburg more patients.

Managing Expectations

Referring physicians want to be informed. Assuming that this is true for your market, define your approach, and then manage what you can provide. Decide what you can do based on the referral volume and strength of your office support team. Focus on practice building, referral development, and competitive challenges. Then, determine what you believe you need to offer.

Next, find out what elements of that plan referring physicians want. For example, some specialists will ask their referral source when they want to hear back from them. It is a great way to let them know you're working to involve them, but only ask if you can implement. A minimum expectations checklist is as follows:

- Initial clinic consult

- Hospitalization

  - Postprocedure

  - Unforeseen change

  - Discharge

- Emergent admission directly to hospital

- Death

- Referral to another specialist—assume you need to unless confirmed otherwise

GENERAL REFERRAL COMMUNICATION PROTOCOLS

Internal dynamics, current relationships, and culture will drive a customized process, but the outline below can offer some parameters.

Timing:

- Call within 24 hours of receiving a hospital referral

- Weekly written correspondence for extended hospital stays; adjust timing based on acuity

- Letter with discharge summary within five days postsurgery or procedure

Accountability:

- Clinic structure will determine the accountability for the communication process— is it led by the physician or by a practice administrator?

- One designated individual should ensure that each communication step is done

- At the end of each week, review the list of cases and their referral sources to be sure that communication has happened

Other Success Factors:

- Let referring physician preference drive communication approach, timing, and tools

- Ask for referral communication preferences when placing a call to a first time referral source

- Be sure the PCP is documented on patient's paperwork upon arrival

- Communicate with all physicians in the referral chain—maintain active communications with other specialists on the case

- Document how referral sources prefer their communication, and stick to that plan

- Hardwire the process into the practice's daily activities

Consistency issues

In most areas of communication, there is optimal, minimal, and somewhere in between. As practices work to define and develop their approach, work on doing a few key things every time. The reason for this suggestion is that often physicians will endorse this need and then craft an approach that is just too intensive to stick with long term. It's better to start small and be consistent—you can always add more touch points later.

When the ball is dropped

It's awful when you have completed a heroic clinical feat, only to get the call that Dr. Smith is unhappy because a patient is back in his office for a follow-up treatment and he has no record of his or her care. Beyond the initial temptation to determine who dropped the ball, all your hard work takes a back seat as you now explain the patient's care and then apologize a couple of times during the call. Even though you hope that by having your minimal consistency plan in place this will not happen, what if it does?

The practice will benefit from having a back-up plan. For example, if they are part of your EMR, ask a staff member to work with them to locate the record. If they are not part of your EMR, make sure a summary sheet can be e-mailed or faxed to them.

One person should manage this at the practice. They also need to have a contact at the hospital. Keep a simple tracking sheet to understand when and why the communication loop was broken—often it is because the right contact name or address was not captured.

Messages Show Value

There are many reasons that peer-to-peer communication matters. Although the first concern is about care delivery, there is more at play. Communication is one of several tools that demonstrate to the referring physician that we value them. It is a tangible demonstration of recognition. For some, that recognition falls closely beside respect. You respect my practice and the relationship with the patient enough to respond to me.

If you are saying, "That is silly, doctors don't really need that," you are likely of the personality type that is not reliant on relationships, or you are surrounded by peers and information exchange with colleagues on a regular basis. But not everyone is. This is about the referring physician and not you. Many referring doctors miss the information exchange with other colleagues, especially if they are not in a practice or geographic area that supports this type of collegiality, whereas referral specialists often have more of it than they want—sort of ironic isn't it? Anyone who has taken any type of personality profile test (e.g., DISC or Myers Briggs) should recognize that relationship and communication are more important to some than to others.

Summary

The survey affirms what readers already assumed: When a physician refers a patient, they expect communication back. Physicians were conservative in the amount of communication they needed. But discharge communication is a must.

The Complete Guide to Physician Relationships

Physicians want to know when a hospitalized patient is discharged because, often, they will be responsible for follow-up care.

There are gaps in what physicians perceive they say and send versus what the recipient believes they receive. The greatest challenge is that everyone is guessing about it. As a result, consistent and standardized communication systems are essential.

Communication among colleagues is likely to change as EMRs make it easier for all caregivers to share in the treatment plan. Does that eliminate the need for those notes that say, "Thank you for allowing me to see Mrs. Doe"? In the near term, those notes are still important. For those physicians who wish to grow their practices through referrals, personal contact is valuable.

What Do Physicians Want to Hear From Marketing?

"The single biggest problem in communication is the illusion that it has taken place."
–George Bernard Shaw

The marketing team is communication central for most organizations and, therefore, is the best tool for connecting all stakeholders—physicians, administrators, marketers, and clinical staff. Because marketing is most closely aligned with the message to consumers through advertising and promotion, often marketers can also quickly provide marketing strategy and implementation with physicians.

This section explores the perception versus reality about communication with physicians. It is important to provide the rationale and reasons behind marketing and communication strategy, rather than just the implementation specifics when you are dealing with scientists—and physicians, at their core, have learned through science.

Successful marketers know that good strategy is built when we understand the needs and wants of our constituents. I asked Daniel Miers, senior vice president, business strategy with Chicago's s|p|m| Marketing & Communications, which specializes in healthcare marketing, to share his thoughts the topic of physicians and marketing. "Propriety suggests: In polite company you should never discuss religion or politics. Add to that guidance, if you want to engage physicians in lively debate, ask them about marketing," he says.

"Depending on the situation, you'll hear it's necessary, it's evil, or maybe it's a necessary evil. Most often, physician opinions of marketing boil down to strong feelings about either what we say, how we say it, or to whom we are saying it," Miers says. "The same holds true in our research of what physicians want to hear from marketing—they have very specific feelings about what they want to hear, how they want to hear it, and to whom they would like marketers to communicate."

As you explore the survey results, more likely than not, it will raise other questions related to your organization and market specifics. Jot them down. Good marketing always starts with research.

How Do Physicians Like to Receive Marketing Information?

The age-old question of "what's the best way to reach physicians with marketing messages?" has become even more complicated. Because of the onslaught of information and messages that physicians receive, it is has never been more challenging to get physicians to read, remember who said what, and respond.

Unfortunately, our survey indicates that there is no single preferred method of communication among physicians (see Figure 7.1). That means, at least in the near term, that marketing teams will continue to grapple with multiple communication methods and formulas.

The Complete Guide to Physician Relationships

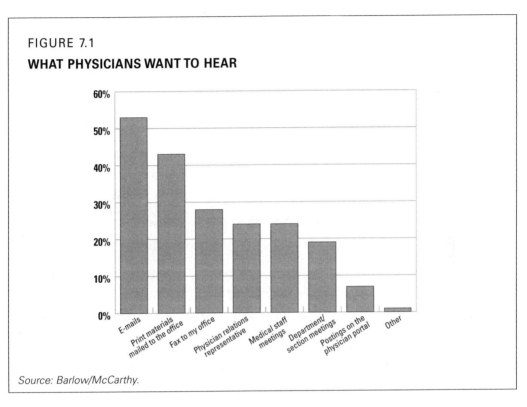

FIGURE 7.1

WHAT PHYSICIANS WANT TO HEAR

Source: Barlow/McCarthy.

Believe it or not, print still seems to be a very desirable tool for the physicians, with 41.6% of respondents preferring to receive printed materials to the office. It ranked second behind e-mail, which was at 50.9%. This is because, in many offices, the handoff to a coordinator or scheduler is often easier than forwarding an e-mail. Plus, a print piece is more mobile and can be tucked away until there's time to read it. And to some, hard copy documents are just more convenient. So the challenge becomes determining what information warrants a printed version and when an e-mail and/or fax works better. Consider printing things that have a longer shelf life or a graph with outcomes data, for example. And e-mail meeting notices or short messages.

According to the survey, the most desired way for physicians to receive updates on programs, services, new physicians, and the organization's plans was via e-mail. That may not be too surprising. But, what perhaps is surprising is that e-mail was the most preferred method of communication for all age groups, except among the very small sample of physicians 65 years old and older.

The survey results did not bode well for physician portals, which only captured 6.4% of the vote. So we have to ask the questions: Is that because of the tool, the type of messages used, or the fact that organizations have not yet leveraged their portals for this purpose? The portal may be an opportunity that has yet to be explored rather than a negative.

Two of the top five communication methods involved a more personal approach. Physicians prefer to receive their information face-to-face, either through individual meetings with a physician relations representative (23.1%) or medical staff (23.1%) and department (17.9%) meetings. This illustrates that personal connection is still important to them.

What This Means for You

In conversations with physicians about communication from hospitals and other providers, one message resonates: relevance. Specifically, physicians want organizations to make the communication that is sent to them more relevant. They report being sent far too much information that does not impact them. For example, a busy OB/GYN recently reported she regularly receives hospital newsletters with updates on processes at the geriatric facility. She shared that managing all the paper—or e-mails—could be a full-time job. Of course it is not. However, as a result, good messages are lost because of the sheer volume.

Own the relevance obligation

Historically, healthcare organizations have been operating under the belief that when it comes to communicating with physicians, more is better. The tendency is to "cover the bases" and make sure they are sent details on everything, just in case. This is not effective. More is simply more. At high-performance institutions, marketing teams carefully scrutinize the message and the target audience. This discipline demonstrates respect for the physician's time, knowledge of their professional specialization, and an understanding of their needs.

Often, the number of departments within an organization sending messages to practices confounds the "relevance" challenge. Marketing can take the lead in facilitating better coordination of these various communication efforts. A useful first step is to audit the current volume of outbound messages, the relevance for the practice, the timing, and overlap (e.g., analyze what you know to be going out and physically tabulate what comes into a specific practice or practices during the same week). This data is the first step in earning the ability to change your approach.

The next step is to find out what doctors need to know. Too often, physicians are not asked what they want or need to know; instead, the marketer "pushes out" a message to the community, with little regard for the physician's needs.

CONSOLIDATING OUTBOUND MESSAGES

Donna Teach, vice president marketing and public relations at Nationwide Children's Hospital in Columbus, completed an audit of their outbound messages and found that community referring physicians were receiving an average of 30+ mailings per month from the free-standing pediatric hospital and research center. The mailings included clinical and business news, updates, and communiqué from numerous departments in the hospital. Content ranged from continuing medical education offerings to new appointment announcements to changes in reference lab protocols. Physicians were burdened to find the content most relevant to them through all the clutter and, as a result, held little value in anything coming from the hospital.

Through interview research with several physician practices, Nationwide Children's learned that physicians found most of the content valuable, but they wanted it consolidated and presented in a format that was easy to sort through. As a result, Nationwide Children's launched their monthly mailing program.

The first step was to centralize the process and eliminate the numerous, separate mailings, says Teach. This was done by restricting access to the medical staff mailing list that was available through the medical staff office. Anyone requesting access to the list was required to state a purpose. If the purpose was an informational mailing, they were directed to the marketing department, where the information could be reviewed and consolidated for inclusion in the packet.

Each packet may include 30 pieces of information, but that information is consolidated into a "briefing report" that can be quickly scanned. The mailing is packaged in a dated folder each month and mailed in an envelope that includes key call-outs of "what's inside." The mailing has been very positively received by both physicians and office staffs, Teach says. Surveys indicate both high value and high retention of the information.

Departments within Nationwide Children's have embraced the mailing because they know it is effective in reaching the physicians. The hospital has explored electronic alternatives for distributing the information, but there has been little interest from the practices—many of whom still prefer the hard copy materials.

Complement your audit with a very succinct, specific survey of physician needs and preferences. Miers at s|p|m| suggests asking the following questions:

- What works here now? What is not working and should be changed or stopped?

- What do other organizations give you (that you value) that we don't?

- What are the top two pieces of information that you need to have right now?

- What behaviors would you likely change right away if you only had the information you require?

Of course, such surveys carry the obligation of follow through. You must close the loop and respond to their top needs. If you can improve relevance and deliver on physicians' most pressing communications needs, you will benefit from better responsiveness and likely save some dollars in exchange for the time spent.

Practice information flow

As practices work to maximize their efficiency, many are working to streamline the information flow. Materials meant for the physician may never reach their eyes if they don't make it through the office screener.

The practice manager can provide great insights into the process they use to filter messages and determine which ones get to the doctor. In practice management meetings, take the opportunity to ask about their process. Determine what they find meaningful, how much time their doctors have to catch up on communication, and what they hear and suggest as the best approach.

As you consider relevance, ask who in the practice needs this. Is it really the doctor, or is it the referral coordinator? Messages that are about access, ease of scheduling, and expanded hours belong in the hands of the referral staff. Calling out the intended audience will enhance the message's impact.

Get print read

Print continues to be a desirable tool for physicians. The fundamental guidelines of creating effective print advertising for consumers apply to communications with physicians, according to Meiers. The following are some best practices:

- **Use simple layouts.** Short, powerful, to-the-point headlines paired with an image that tells the story quickly.

- **Keep body copy legible.** Avoid large blocks of intimidating copy (i.e., easier to ignore than to read), hard-to-read fonts, and designs that place copy over pictures that hamper readability.

- **Go with the flow.** In English, we read from top left to bottom right; don't fight those tendencies.

- **Answer the question, "What's in it for me?"** Make the benefit to the physician clear and obvious. And be sure that the benefit offered is a benefit the physician needs or can appreciate.

As physicians become less visible within the walls of our organizations, because of hospitalist-type programs, getting information about the hospital out to them can be critical to engagement. Ann Maloley, our lead in practice marketing at Barlow/McCarthy, says physicians appreciate knowing about any clinical or operational developments at the hospital that may affect the efficiency or effectiveness of their work. Additionally, if there are new developments that may affect their patients' experiences or may be related to access or service, that's important information for them as well.

Based on her conversations with practice managers and physicians within their own practices, Maloley stresses the importance of fact- and data-based content. They don't much have time for "soft" news and prefer news that can help them with their own practice development—for example, new clinical studies, changes in payer relations, the addition of a physician-only access line for referrals and consults. Messages need to focus on "them," not "us."

Visual consistency is important with any print materials, including materials for physicians. A standard masthead and consistent graphics can help the materials stand out as "official" documents. It should look clinical and informative, not slick and glitzy.

Where there is opportunity, consider supporting specialty-to-specialty communications. Look for ways to communicate clinical information that help physicians familiarize themselves with each other and the clinical expertise being offered at the organization. This type of communication takes on a more educational feel.

In addition, physicians prefer learning about a facility's clinical capabilities through clinical education, according to Maloley.

Avoid e-mail abuse

Just as e-mail is easy to create and easy to send—especially to very large distribution lists—it can become easy to avoid and ignore. One clinician revealed it was not uncommon to receive 30 to 50 e-mail communications by Tuesday afternoon. People tire of electronic communication quickly and they will master the ways to sort messages by sender and mass delete offending (unread) e-mail.

Quote docs

Kathy Dean, marketing director with OHSU in Portland, OR, shared with me that it is great to see more physicians open to e-mail communications. "It allows us to do so much more than just deliver information. It allows us to more easily target who we send to, track who is reading what, and also provide two-way communication with the physician," she says.

But, to do it right, you must first understand that e-communication is about more than just taking print pieces and pasting them into e-mails, says Dean. "E-mail is usually scanned, not read. Short headlines with links for more information will have better readership than lengthy paragraphs of text copy. A click on a link can bring the physician to a portal or a blog where they may find more info, or leave a comment. Regardless of the delivery method, the key to communications with physicians is to stay focused on delivering the information they need in an easily accessible way."

David Shipley and Will Schwalbe provide good advice on effectively using the e-mail in their 2007 book *Send: The Essential Guide to Email for Office and Home*. The following are some guidelines and cautionary notes:

- The ease of e-mail encourages unnecessary exchanges. Make sure that the information is essential to this physician.

- E-mail has largely replaced the phone call, but not every phone call should be replaced.

- You can reach almost everyone, but don't assume instant/inappropriate familiarity.

- The fact that e-mail defies time zones also means that it can defy propriety. Every e-mail is an interruption. If the matter isn't urgent, other communications can be more appropriate and less intrusive.

- The ease with which an e-mail can be forwarded poses a danger. Assume that everything you write will be forwarded.

- E-mail attachments don't just come with baggage; they *are* baggage. If every e-mail is an interruption, every attachment is an additional burden.

Face-to-face

Physicians still feel more involved when there is personal communication. Consider all venues, including meetings, social activities, visits to the practice, and educational opportunities that allow for that personal exchange of ideas. While reading this, I suspect that teams across the country are saying, "Ours won't come!" My only come back is to say, "Keep trying." Consider face-to-face connections that add value for the physician at a personal or business level. Find messages that help them beyond getting what you need. There is no magic formula to make this work—test times, methods, and messages until you find a formula that will work for your environment.

COMMONSENSE E-MAIL FOR DOCTORS ... AND OTHERS!

1. Sell it in. If e-mail is used as a communications tool, then introduce the plan to the doctors. Let them know what to expect via e-mail, share who the sender will be, and outline the frequency. Sell it in!

2. Index it. "Indexed" headlines let the doctor quickly scan for desired information.

3. Coordinate, don't spray. Manage the frequency of sending relevant information.

4. Central dispatcher. E-mails should come from one alias e-mail to show it's from the hospital.

5. Test it. Conduct a survey a few months after launch to ask whether the information is helpful and useful; adjust as necessary.

6. Just the facts. Although it's necessary to make the e-mail look attractive and eye-catching, the idea is to get them to read it and find it useful. So be sure your e-mails are clean and uncluttered, with minimal graphics.

7. Multiple methods. Print materials should be sent to the clinic manager because the doctor receives so much mail that it could get lost in shuffle; include information helpful to the clinic manager; faxes should be the same way.

Physician representatives deliver depth

Another interesting finding from the study was the desire for visits with physician representatives. Although, this is a useful means of communication overall physicians in the 45 to 64 age group indicated they especially appreciated these resources. One possible explanation is that physicians in this age range are the busiest. For them, focused problem-solution conversations are essential and preferred over wading through e-mail or printed materials.

The promise of portals remains unrealized

It is impossible to know at this time whether the portal may still represent an opportunity rather than a negative. However, communicators should be cautious about adding yet another "source to keep track of" to the physician's communications load—especially if use of the portal is not fully integrated into the physician's practice habits. As this medium matures, communicators should consider whether certain types of messages are better suited to the portal, and then study the best visual and creative means to present them. Quite possibly, the portal may be the best platform for timely clinical communications, such as H1N1 protocols, emergency department diversion updates, and disaster preparedness information.

Some organizations are currently providing patient information through a portal that physicians can access, so the foundation may already be in place. When the time is right to add a portal to your communication toolkit, getting buy-in up front will be important. Understand what kind of information physicians would like to access through a portal, be sure their technology is compatible with your system, and provide education to help access and navigate the portal efficiently.

Opportunity for Action

It is easy to become a creature of habit—do a group e-mail or a fax blast or create a one-page fact sheet—just because we have the tools and we are working to check it off the list. That's what happens to us when we are reacting to demands. But there is an opportunity to be more proactive and plan ahead for those messages we know need to be delivered. It requires going one step deeper in our physician marketing strategy, but that ability to determine type of message and type of medium could help bring balance to the marketing communication plan. The plan then takes on additional value if we build in the other departments and their monthly communications. Assuming that you have done the audit and earned buy-in for a more effective communications approach with physicians, the next step is consistent implementation. Consider a simple process that will assist you in determining the market, the relevance, the tool, and the time frame.

Here's a checklist to get you started:

- Determine your overall physician communication strategy: key topics, audience segments, and desired outcomes.

- Learn the nuances of each practice or practices by category: understand their communication expectations and needs based on predetermined criteria such as specialty, relationship with the hospital, and age of the practice.

- Advocate the need for marketing to manage messages from all areas within the organization in order to organize and streamline the flow of information.

- Develop a process for gathering meaningful content, writing relevant messages, determining most suitable tools, and setting distribution schedules.

- Standardize a layout and visual elements to be sure physicians will want to read the material.

- Measure activity to learn what messages and mediums drives response and action. Modify the plan accordingly.

There will always be other little things that pop up. Having a system with protocols and methodology in place can certainly help you streamline the process.

Summary

Relevance, balance, and options are the standout obligations when we consider the best marketing communication for physicians. Although it would streamline the process and save dollars, this research—and our own experience—will validate that we need to have a full toolkit of choices for communication.

Plan ahead so you are sure to stay in touch with this audience. That's what marketers do with any other audience, right? Be prepared for shifts in need and expectations. As practices are adjusting to the changing times, the information they need will likely adjust. As marketers, it's our job to prepare for those times and redesign our strategy accordingly. No doubt other facilities are communicating with these offices as well, so we have to be sure that our communications serve a purpose for them and demonstrate our desire to share and support.

As we test approach and impact, we'll do well to remember which type of tool worked the best for a specific message and group of physicians. If ever you get to that flat response, it's time to review and retool!

Promoting Services

There is often a constant knock on the door of the vice president of marketing's office from a physician who says, "I need a billboard to promote the new robot," or whatever their specialty may be. We have often categorized this behavior as self-promotion. And although there may be some self-promotion, physicians clearly believe that mass marketing grows business. Additionally, physicians want to be associated with a strong brand. As a stakeholder in the organization, they feel proud (or not proud, as the case may be) when their organization is in the spotlight. Many physicians would tell you that mass marketing is necessary to stay competitive. So it makes sense that they view exposure in media as the No. 1 way to promote services (see Figure 8.1) and want to see TV ads and billboards featuring their hospital partner.

Physicians rated grassroots efforts that connect with other physicians as the second best way to promote services. Although some physicians are much better at this than others, organizations will benefit when they are able to provide a framework and streamlined process for physician-to-physician marketing. The good news about the high response rate (36.2%) is that almost as many physicians who believe mass marketing is necessary recognize that business comes directly from other doctors.

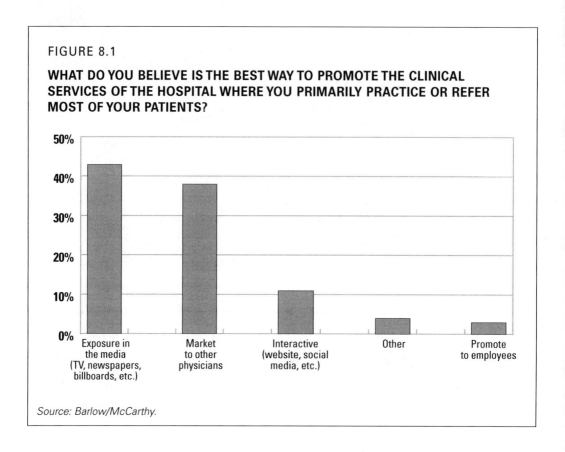

FIGURE 8.1

WHAT DO YOU BELIEVE IS THE BEST WAY TO PROMOTE THE CLINICAL SERVICES OF THE HOSPITAL WHERE YOU PRIMARILY PRACTICE OR REFER MOST OF YOUR PATIENTS?

Source: Barlow/McCarthy.

When looking at whether age plays a role in what physicians view as the best way to promote services, there is some evidence that suggests younger doctors may be more interested in marketing to other physicians, whereas there is a tendency for older physicians to prefer mass advertising. However, the survey sample size was too small to provide a strong assertion.

Interactive media commands about 11% of the vote. Although there were slightly more physicians who recognized this in the younger age group, there were doctors in every age group who recognized this as a valuable marketing tool. With a marketplace that is so reliant on interactive media, this percentage will only continue to grow.

Not surprising, but a bit disappointing, is the fact that physicians skipped over employees. Astute marketers recognize that employees can be some of the best brand ambassadors for the organization. The takeaway here may be that employees are currently not being empowered as brand ambassadors, so perhaps the responsibility lies with marketers to encourage staff to promote the brand. If physicians see that the staff is engaged in promoting the organization to patients and the community, they likely will see the value in promoting to employees as well.

Managing Our 'We Know Best' Attitude

Organizations should follow the lead of the people with the most expertise, but it is an uphill battle for marketing. You've heard it before: Everyone thinks they are a marketer. This research indicates that if marketers really do know best and have the best expertise, they still have a ways to go in educating our doctors about it because most marketers do not support mass media for promotion of specialized healthcare services. There are fabulous marketers in healthcare facilities, yet I am not certain that there are fabulous internal plans to demonstrate expertise in media selection with good data and involved physicians. Moving forward, this can be formalized so physicians are able to understand the marketing mix that is selected. Physicians appreciate data that shows the medium selected and the results achieved. If your organization needs physicians to support a range of marketing tools, then educate them about the approach using data.

Marketing to physicians—our job or theirs?

Given the high percentages of physicians who understand the value of marketing to other physicians, we have to determine whether they see that as the marketers' job or theirs. Many specialists, perhaps more so in prestigious academic medical centers, believe that the creation of a brochure that shows who is in the department will be adequate in creating awareness and growing business. But field representatives will tell you that the brochures rarely get opened. On many occasions, I have heard the comment, "I wish they would quit spending money on all this slick material and just get me a discharge summary."

If you are challenged to determine what works for marketing to physicians, test the marketing approaches with your prospective referral sources and then use the data you gather to position stronger physician-to-physician connections.

Hitting your stride

Many cutting edge marketing leaders have refocused resources to address the physician-as-customer strategy. The findings in this survey (see Figure 8.1) give ample fodder for establishing better methods to let them know all that marketing can do.

For example, the survey did not ask about physicians' current perceptions of marketing. But it is an interesting thought, and a survey could ask the following questions:

- How do you define marketing?

- How does the process at your primary facility support physician connections with the community and with other doctors?

- What has been your role in working with the marketing team?

- If marketing were able to help you refine your messages for any audience, where would you like the help?

- What role if any would you like to play in the future?

As a marketing team, speculate for a minute on what you think the answers might be and then detail what you wish them to be. If the medical staff has done more sabotage than support, the marketing team can take some steps to further demonstrate credibility. Consider involving those physicians in the marketing process when clinical expertise is needed. Let them hear the marketing discussion of strategy and approach for determining the best communications vehicles.

Basic brain stuff

Many marketers cut their teeth in the consumer world. Understanding consumer behavior is an important link to effective marketing. Even though physicians are consumers, the marketers who are the most effective in working with physicians have adapted their consumer approach to physicians. By understanding the role of the physician better, they have created a special approach for working closely with them. Think about it: Most of the time, the patient tells the doctor what is wrong and the doctor asks questions ruling out different conditions, then defines the problem and makes a recommendation. Marketers are more effective when they bring forward a need, offer options and discussion of process, and then jointly reach a decision. Physicians will most likely have ideas of their own, so providing options, the rationale behind them, and even a recommendation is much better than leaving the options and choices up to them.

PRIORITIZE YOUR MARKETING STRATEGY

Chris Bevolo, owner of the Minneapolis-based agency Interval and a nationally recognized thought leader in healthcare marketing, shared the following thoughts on promoting services and the survey results.

"The results are not surprising, but still disappointing. The good news is that I would have imagined the number of physicians who rated mass advertising as the best way to promote services to be much higher. The bad news is that at 40%, it's still the highest rated response, rated higher than two potentially more potent strategies—interactive and marketing to other physicians."

The truth, says Bevolo, is that all of these approaches will be needed at some level to maximize marketing efforts. But there should be a hierarchy of strategies, starting with those considered fundamental in nature. For example, no matter what else a hospital does, they must have a comprehensive, clear, and compelling website in place, as the Internet is typically the first place consumers will go to learn about an organization's offerings. It also provides one of the best calls-to-action of any hospital marketing effort.

"Before you go out knocking on doors with direct marketing or mass advertising, you better be ready for those audiences to come back to you, and that starts with having a solid website," says Bevolo.

Then, knowing the crucial role physician referrals play in driving volumes, having a robust physician sales and communications program would be next in line. This brings up another key concern for Bevolo when analyzing the responses.

"Only one physician responded with 'word of mouth' (which shows up under the 'Other' category), and according to many experts and much research, word of mouth

The Complete Guide to Physician Relationships

PRIORITIZE YOUR MARKETING STRATEGY (CONT.)

is the number one driver of consumer decision-making, even beyond physician referral and insurance," says Bevolo. "The key to driving word of mouth, of course, is delivering an exceptional patient experience. The point is that if you offer the best service around, much of your marketing takes care of itself. Look at Mayo Clinic or Starbucks for that matter. Both of these organizations developed world-leading brands without any promotional marketing or advertising. That's because of the experience they delivered."

The challenge this survey question reveals, says Bevolo, is that most physicians have these priorities backward, ranking mass advertising ahead of patient experience development, interactive, and physician-oriented strategies.

"The goal of a hospital marketer should be to help educate his or her physicians on the benefits and priority of various marketing strategies, and to clearly articulate both the expense and the limitations of mass advertising to drive volumes. Only after other, more foundational, strategies are taken care of should a hospital consider stepping up in a significant way with paid media campaigns."

It is also important to tell them up front what you need them to do. For example, before they review marketing materials, explain that everyone writes in their own style and that you are confident with the language. Explain that the area you need the physician to explore is the clinical content and phrases to describe the service. The idea is to distinguish your MD as marketing director from their MD as medical doctor in an effort to set boundaries of responsibilities.

Active Support of Physician-to-Physician Connections

Many organizations are becoming more serious about helping physicians connect to their peers. Throughout the survey, we have found that this is a critical element in enhancing referral relationships. The first question to ask is, "Are all connections created equal?" For instance, do we get the same impact from physicians talking at a medical staff meeting as we do with doing howdy rounds with a rep driving the physician from practice to practice, or attending an education program, or an informal discussion? Clearly the answer is no, so if organizations are investing in programs that are reliant on physicians, there is an opportunity to get more serious about maximizing their success in this regard.

Just because physicians believe it is important and effective does not mean that they know which approaches will maximize the effectiveness. Medical school is a wonderful place for collegial work, but the groups and support teams of colleagues are predetermined. It rarely occurs to many physicians that they will need to work to earn the environment that supports their referral base. Once again, we can have success through education and sharing of possible approaches and then demonstrating the impact.

Better than howdy rounds

Formal physician relations programs can do a great job of creating physician-to-physician connections. But let's first talk about "howdy rounds." Leverage your program to get more strategic than just dropping in with a doctor to say hello. It is far more effective to speak with the prospective referral source prior to the meeting, to gain insights into their needs in the specialty area, and then to stage a brief meeting with the physician. The rep can then follow up after the meeting to determine effectiveness and speak with the office team to provide details for the referral process.

Education for practice building and referral relations

Many organizations offer education programs to physicians who are interested in building their practices. A portion of the curriculum is about physician-to-physician connections. Simple process steps, such as creating name tags, assigning staff to introduce new participants, or having a physician relations rep to welcome attendees can be very effective in creating the right environment for one physician to get acquainted with his or her peer group. Of note, these continuing medical education programs are both effective and welcomed by doctors.

Do we have to?

For some physicians, there is a bit of a stigma about needing to be visible and create conversations that position expertise and grow referrals. This is old school thinking that does not hold up today. As the survey affirms (36% of physicians say the best way to grow the practice is through other physicians), physicians like to work with colleagues they know. In reality, personal connections encourage better communication, and we know that better communication leads to better patient experience and quality of care that is delivered.

If you have a medical staff that seems reluctant, evaluate their reason. Some are so introverted that this exercise is just exhausting. If that is the case, have the physician relations team find small group settings to make it more palatable. At the end of the day, some physicians struggle with face-to-face meetings. In those rare cases where no setting really works, consider an article written by the physician with a phone call or a personal note. Connections are essential for those who are hoping to earn referrals.

Referrals based on organization brand

There are a handful of organizations that generate referrals simply because of the organization's brand—not necessarily because of personal connections. Although many wish to be recognized by their name, some are not. Or, the name is there but the pull is not strong enough to drive referrals.

For those organizations that have the distinction of receiving referrals based on brand identity, it's because many individuals worked hard to get that brand recognition and created the personal relationships that got it all started. The success of these centers does not detract at all from the obligation to have personal connections. It is interesting to note that in conversations with doctors who refer to these entities, they will often say, "I refer to Mayo or one of the others." If the subsequent question is "to whom?," they will give a physician's name.

SUPPORTING PHYSICIAN-TO-PHYSICIAN CONNECTIONS

Here is a checklist organizations should consider when working behind the scenes to support physician-to-physician connectivity.

1. Formalize onboarding activities for new recruits and your process of connecting the new physicians with potential referral sources.

   a. Employed practices should understand their role in referral development before the physician's contract is signed.

   b. Proactively work with your private practice offices, too. Do not assume that a senior partner will take the time to do this. Sometimes their referral source is not a fit for the new colleague.

2. Prioritize by selecting the specialties that align with specialties highlighted for business growth.

3. Create times for introduction at meetings with a streamlined process to ensure those who need to meet others are afforded that opportunity.

4. Offer educational sessions on topics like practice development and referral management.

5. Connect primary care and specialists. They need each other, and yet they are often not on the same page in terms of expectations.

6. Support the face-to-face interactions with appropriate printed materials, such as clinical briefs and specialty fact sheets.

7. Work behind the scenes with the practice manager to get their support and buy-in into the process; point out the benefits of these actions.

8. Create accountability in the plan to increase success.

Word of caution

With all of this momentum behind physician-to-physician connections, keep in mind the possible pitfall of establishing these personal relationships: what if the physician leaves your organization and, worse yet, moves to a competitor? Although I am a fervent supporter of developing physician relations, I ask you to keep this in mind. When you're helping to develop these relationships, be sure that you're planting seeds of the deeper clinical expertise within the specialty that physician represents and, when possible, extend the relationship to more than one specialist within the clinical service line.

Social Media and Web Innovations

How many times a day do you go to the Web to look something up? Whether it is a Facebook® account, an address for a restaurant, or background on a consulting firm you intend to use, all of our tools are programmed for immediate access. Today's medical students are wired to use their phones for schedules, medications, and care delivery. It has made research much easier, but it also means that our Web identity must be current, create rapport with the audience we intend, and have back-end connections that will ensure responsiveness.

Impact of social media

Hospitals are working to define their applications for the many social media tools that are part of everyday life for many consumers. Physicians are also following social media trends, but many are still in a wait-and-see mode. But Facebook, YouTube, Twitter, and blogs are attracting tremendous attention. The key question is what role these tools can play in positioning physician expertise and whether it will have the desired impact.

- Lee Aase, director of the Center for Social Media at Mayo Clinic, shared his view on the potential impact of YouTube with the following examples:

  - A YouTube video by a hematology/oncology physician on the topic of myelofibrosis resulted in more than 50 new patients—one of whom was from Greece.

  - A Mayo surgeon created a YouTube video on pectus excavatum. She reports more than 30 new patients.

Although these are niche areas, which make the tracking a bit cleaner, it shows the power of personal search. Aase says that when good information is provided on YouTube, you are able to create a bond with consumers, and patients follow.

Patients searching for information about their disease often find support groups, which also share information on videos and blogs. It is all about information, and the social media tools tend to lead patients from one to the other. You create a blog with an embedded video that can include links, and then you tweet the link.

Interest in social media tools is not limited to a certain segment of the medical staff, says Aase. Even though younger physicians at Mayo are more comfortable with the applications, Aase says there has been good internal interest and a spirit of inquiry across the board.

Don't neglect your hospital's website

The hospital's website is about hospital services, but prospective patients will expect to find ample detail about the physicians who have privileges at that hospital. They don't separate us. And they tend to judge our quality by how the website looks and how easy it is to navigate. If I were a patient considering a knee replacement and I went to your website, would I easily find the service capabilities and choices of orthopedic surgeons on staff? Much of this is basic Web development that no doubt is already on your marketing radar, but I believe it's worthy of a mention.

Proud physicians want us to share extensive background and education details on the Web. I have read—okay, tried to read—through these bios. Find a better way. Again, it starts with education to the doctors about best practices, what gets read, and what your Web strategy will accomplish for them. A few lines about education and a bit more about the patients they treat will go much further.

Make sure that your physician-focused Web messages are consistent with other messages they hear or share. Doctors—again, back to their training and the way they are wired—pick at every single potential discrepancy. Find those discrepancies before they do and engage them in your Web strategy—the background behind the decision, the process used, and the areas where you had to compromise. It would be great if we could move them in the direction of referring their patients to our website. But that all starts with their confidence in our content and a bit of pride in association.

Employed physician website

Many organizations struggle with the best Web strategy for their employed practices. Historically, many opted to provide connectivity to the practices via a link on the health system's website. If you have gone that route, it may be time to test ease of use, finding the practice and brand association with your target audience. In the race for having the practice feel that the hospital understands their needs and markets for them, their own website comes up first in every conversation.

Summary

This research affirms that the physician is very much a consumer and believes that telling others about services through media is the best approach. As hospital marketers make choices about their marketing methods, it will be important to involve physicians in discussions about marketing objectives, media selection methodology, and results to the bottom line—including theirs. This dialogue is important if we want them to understand and support the media strategy decisions.

Physicians recognize that marketing to other physicians can be very effective in creating awareness. As hospital marketers, it is important to spell out the type of marketing that can be most impactful for other physicians. This generally requires conversations about personal connectivity rather than mass mailings to the physician office. Physicians are bright and most do this very well, but we cannot assume that they have the experience or marketing expertise to initiate. Physician relations, education, and medical staff connections can play a strong role in success.

Social media marketing is front and center as we explore new ways to streamline communication with the most relevant audiences. Most physicians are tech savvy and will prefer early involvement in these tools. This assumes that we make it easy for them.

Bottom line as it relates to this discussion: Physicians want to be aligned with a strong partner, and they want to be busy. Marketing can help them with both—it's a matter of open dialogue, a bit of education, and a clear understanding of best practice actions that can show results.

Supporting Specialists

When determining where to refer patients, primary care providers prefer a face-to-face interaction to learn about clinical expertise 75% of the time (see Figure 9.1). This speaks volumes about their appreciation for dialogue on clinical topics. Meetings with the specialists were preferred by 45% of the survey respondents. Physician relations representatives/liaisons fulfill an important role and were the desired approach by 28.5% of physicians. Continuing medical education (CME) has a role to play in informing the primary care audience about expertise, but it was the preferred method by just 10%. Mailings and directories scored the same, with 8% of the survey participants indicating that this was their preferred method of learning about expertise and services provided.

Talk Is Not Cheap

It is a constant battle for physicians to balance clinical time with the other duties of growing a practice. Doctors are quick to point out that if they are not taking care of patients, they are not getting paid. Even those who are employed get compensated based on the number of patients they treat. Because time is money, some specialists question the value of taking time to meet with other physicians to discuss their clinical area of expertise. Many practice administrators are quick to suggest that the primary care physicians (PCP) don't have time for these conversations either. But, according to the physicians who answered our survey, it is clear that they feel that face-to-face conversations are valued.

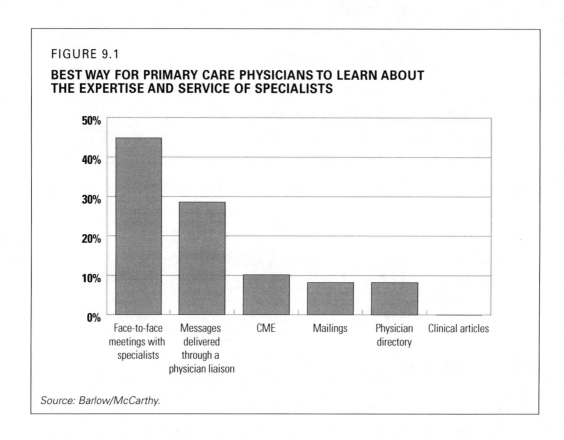

FIGURE 9.1

BEST WAY FOR PRIMARY CARE PHYSICIANS TO LEARN ABOUT THE EXPERTISE AND SERVICE OF SPECIALISTS

Source: Barlow/McCarthy.

If you have specialists who are reluctant to implement personal meetings, assuming that they have the right aptitude for this, commit to demonstrating the impact. A discussion with the specialist will help you understand their reluctance. First, you should make certain that there is interest in expanding their practice. This may be overall volume or a specific procedure that they would like to grow or a select geographic area. If they have no interest in additional growth of any type in their practice, it's hard to create any measurable need for doing face-to-face meetings.

Staging physician-to-physician meetings

The last chapter offered suggestions to encourage specialists to initiate meetings with their peers. In most markets today, the hospital stands ready and willing to support this effort—assuming that the physician is willing.

"We have found that specialist–primary care physician communications is the basis for the strongest, most lasting relationships. Face-to-face visits and phone conversations are always the preferred route, but time is valuable and it's often difficult to bring PCPs and specialists together," Susan M. Alcorn, chief communications officer for Geisinger Health System in Danville, PA.

Physician liaisons can play a key role here. The physician liaison should develop comprehensive plans that will help prioritize visits, eliminate duplication, and identify influential staff members and preferred communication methods, Alcorn says. "The bottom line: Be strategic, make sure every visit and contact counts, and be respectful of each physician's time and preferences."

MAKING PHYSICIAN-TO-PHYSICIAN MEETINGS WORK

1. Fine-tune the presentation

   - Consider having a simple sheet of tips from other physicians about what they liked or what they did not.

   - Make sure that the specialist creates a climate of sharing. Lectures just will not have the same impact as dialogue.

   - Assess and then support the physician in making their services/expertise appealing. Consider tools or stories or data as needed. (Some of their topics are important but lack in those elements that just draw you in.)

2. Practice background

   - Make certain that the specialist knows whether this physician has referred to them, their practice, or your organization.

   - Understand their market, including patient base, payer, local healthcare providers, and history.

   - Personal background about where they trained and how long they have been in the community is helpful.

   - Offer insights on their demeanor and expectations. If this physician is all about the data and outcomes, a different approach would be needed than if they were about relationships and getting to know the doctor at a more personal level.

   - This is the point where you make certain to discuss the importance of "not talking down" to those who have not trained in the specialty.

3. Make good choices about who to see

   - Use data to determine which markets make the most sense. Prepare rationale because, more often than not, the specialist will have an opinion in this area.

MAKING PHYSICIAN-TO-PHYSICIAN MEETINGS WORK (CONT.)

- Keep the list small so you can be sure they have good follow-up in place.

- Allow the specialist to understand that the practice may want to discuss and refer more than just the niche area they hope to grow. Discuss it so they are aware of the implications. The referral source treats all, so they expect their specialist to have the same approach, regardless of payer or other criteria.

4. Set realistic expectations

- Determine what the specialist hopes to achieve as a result of their efforts. Once learned, offer alternatives if you feel that they are too aggressive. Discuss the referral cycle, and remind them that the doctor may not have their type of case every week.

- Affirm that goodwill does not always have an immediate return. Help them grow a little patience if this is new and uncomfortable.

- Assure the specialist that you will stay in touch with the physicians and continue to look for opportunities for future visits and to strengthen the relationship.

5. Follow up and continue the conversation

- The physician relations rep/liaison can visit the practice a week or so after the meeting to learn what the practice thought. Feedback needs to be shared with the physician, including positives that encourage subsequent visits and recommendations for how to finesse areas that need attention.

- Encourage the practice to measure new referrals, but be sure that the time frames are generous. Remind them that it often takes a little time to have the right patient to refer.

- Keep the topic present in the target physician's mind by augmenting the initial conversation with supplemental information—data, journal articles on the subject, or perhaps a second visit from a clinical director.

If the specialists indicate an interest in growing their practice or service area, but time away from the practice or the drain on personal time is a huge concern, then learn more about their best times to be away. Determine several options, and then the physician relations/liaison can work to accommodate their schedule. This is never a perfect science, but it is much better to clarify what they desire at the onset.

Saving gas

If the physician is very limited on time, presentations to a group—either live or via a personal practice webinar—can be a good alternative. For personal presentations, make sure that the primary care physician's specific topic of interest is determined before the meeting. Again, a liaison can visit the practice in the weeks prior and speak to one or two physicians to learn what topics may be of most interest. This enhances the engagement during the presentation and encourages a stronger dialogue.

To be successful with these "exclusive webinars" keep the following criteria in mind:

- Make it feel personal by setting up the webinar in the primary care practice so the atmosphere allows for shared dialogue throughout the presentation.

- The webinar needs to be more than a lecture with PowerPoint® slides.

- If you have some very interesting technology, use the slides to share clinical applications.

- Consider having the representative from the specialist's organization travel to the primary care group. With this approach there is an assurance that the technology is in place, and the representative can also personally gauge the reaction from the audience.

- Schedule 20–30 minutes for presentation, with time for questions and discussion.

Although webinars can work nicely for creating general awareness, they are especially valuable if the PCP has had or currently has a patient who may be a candidate for the procedure being discussed.

Facilitating clinical discussions

Keeping up with advances in technology, clinical protocols, and new drugs can be a full-time job. It is important for physicians who are subspecialized to constantly connect with their peers to understand innovations, changes in protocol, and different techniques. The literature is overwhelming. In addition, PCPs will never understand the specialty areas with the same breadth and depth—nor do they really want to.

As specialists work to earn referrals, it is important that they commit to a conversation that starts with the needs of that PCP. Although they may be fascinated by some of the new technology or impressed with the impact of a new protocol, this conversation needs to start with an appreciation of the type of symptoms that a patient will present, the early tests that will indicate a concern, the techniques that will help rule out other conditions, and the recommended time frame for a referral. Most importantly, the PCP is interested in learning about how to manage those specific patients in their clinic and when the appropriate time is to send them to the specialist. Explain the PCP's need with the specialist to maximize the experience for both doctors.

Data is always a wonderful tool for discussion as well. If the specialist wants to bring anything along, the recommendation is either an article or abstract they recently published or summary data findings on quality, outcomes, or service.

The right relations message

In many organizations, at least a portion of the specialist meetings are coordinated by the physician relations staff. So it is important that the rep understands the strategic areas that are ready for growth and that they have systems of follow through and commitment from the specialists before there is commitment to "get in the car" and offer a specialist meeting. As physicians' practice time becomes more precious, the intensity of the gatekeeper screening increases. There needs to be clarity regarding the reason for the visit, and the visit needs to address the practice's "what's in it for me?" view.

These specialist meetings are more productive and, ultimately, more successful if the rep/liaison has developed an initial connection with the targeted practices. The specialist meeting often represents one stage in the sales process that should take place—after a general rapport has been developed with the clinic physicians and staff and conversations have uncovered practice details, referral preferences, and clinical needs. Then the stage has been set to bring the specialist into a comfortable and welcoming environment, open to having the conversation. This is when you initiate steps 1 and 2 from the checklist.

Avoid Only One Option

Even though the survey asked doctors to give us just one choice regarding their referral preferences, every marketer who reads this will recognize that multiple methods of communication are a necessity—not an option. In most markets, it is physically and financially impossible to have personal meetings with every doctor about all the specialists and the services they provide. Targeted marketing plans consider the key audiences and communication objectives. Then look at the appropriate tools to effectively carry the message. For those practices that may not accept personal visits, a separate plan should be in place that offers more mailings, invitations, education, or other tools.

Your communications mix will likely include print materials. Many marketers seem to intuitively know what type of content is appropriate for the various audiences they communicate with. It's important to note the importance of managing content in print materials for physicians—from direct mail pieces and event invitations, from clinical articles to education schedules—the focus should be brief, factual, and clean.

The directory continues to be a source of discussion for many facilities. Although it is not a driver for referral selection, it does streamline access for referral coordinators—and that's a good thing. Whether it needs to be print or online is best answered by the facility depending on their market. Across the country, the trend for larger facilities is to shift to an online directory to manage accuracy with frequent updates. If your facility is working through the decision to print, consider a simple survey with the referral coordinators in your market.

Education Beyond CME

Education is just that, and CME is not a marketing tool. Having said that, the opportunity for specialists to present learnings in their field of expertise is a wise decision. Beyond the educational value, this tool sets up opportunities for face-to-face connection. CME is also a strong positioning strategy—the ability to educate connotes expertise.

If your organization offers CME, facilitate the personal connections by encouraging introductions. Physician relations teams can also support your efforts by learning about topics of interest in the market. Work with your education department on topics, target lists, and methods of promotion.

Organizations are getting creative in the way they offer educational programs—if it seems unreasonable to ask physicians to drive to your facility for a session, consider offering Web-based presentations, or take the presentation to them. Set up in a neighboring community hospital and invite the surrounding physicians. It's convenient for them, it's on their turf, and it can send a message of goodwill, too.

As marketers, consider the look of your invitations and the look of other educational and social events. Make certain that the brand is clear and consistent. The desire is to have visual recognition that is physician-focused.

The Complete Guide to Physician Relationships

Summary

Studies show that PCPs continue to have a strong influence over the choice of specialist for the majority of tertiary referrals. Although some specialists would like to believe that marketing communications, education, or directory listings will be effective referral generators, our survey affirms the need to go further. Creating opportunities to connect physicians is best done through a coordinated effort, and that generally falls to the facility that offers the services. Beyond that, specialists must be willing. This includes creating the right approach, follow up, and willingness to recognize the importance of the relationship.

It is not a one size fits all. The ability to support connections through tools, education, and ongoing awareness is just part of the marketing process. Marketing and physician relations staff teams are in a great position to support this effort. The skills of these individuals combined with the clinical cachet carried by the specialists create a powerful combination.

What Do Physicians Want to Hear From Physician Relations?

"To listen well is a powerful means of communication."
–John Marshall

Physician relations is now an essential part of the hospital–physician toolkit as an accepted approach for organizations to communicate with those physicians who have the potential to refer and admit to their organization. For our purposes, it is the use of representatives for face-to-face relationship building, usually with the intent of earning new referrals. It has been very effective—referrals can be measured, issues are uncovered, and intelligence is shared with leadership. In an era where messages are everywhere, a physician relations representative has an ideal opportunity to be relevant.

Organizations love the fact that business growth can be directly attributed to these conversations with the representative. Leaders and physician specialists are able to rely on the representative to connect them with the right physicians. Having representation regularly going into the practice gives solid intelligence about how the practices are doing, what competitive threats exist, how practices perceive the hospital, and how referral decisions are made. There are many benefits to the organization, but do the physicians feel the same way?

Recently, the market has been bombarded with reps of all types who want a few minutes of the doctor's time. For every rep that is well prepared and sensitive to the needs of the practice, there seems to be one that is there to push products and drive their own agenda. This has changed the market dynamics for physician relations. Now much more time and effort is spent just getting in the door. The practices are weary and struggle to decide "who gets in." Would you make the cut?

We know that best practice programs show solid referral gains for the organization. But what is the perception of value for the doctor, and do they feel that this type of communication is helpful? The survey was designed to uncover the physician relations rep's perceived value but also to determine what physicians envision the role to be. The third objective was to determine whether specialists felt that the physician relations rep was effective as a practice builder for them. Physician relations reps do offer value, but there is some work to be done (see Figure 10.1).

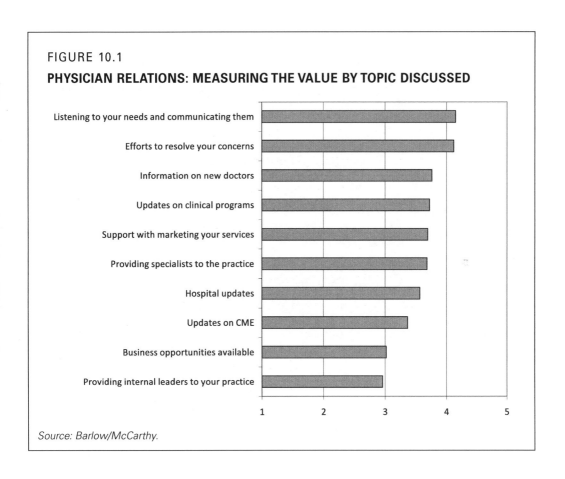

FIGURE 10.1

PHYSICIAN RELATIONS: MEASURING THE VALUE BY TOPIC DISCUSSED

Source: Barlow/McCarthy.

Measuring the Value

Scoring on a five-point scale is a great way to determine comparative value as we seek to understand how the physician relations activities are perceived by the doctors.

The area that doctors say is of most help is listening to their needs and communicating with them, which scored 4.15 out of 5. This is followed closely by efforts to resolve concerns, which says that doctors value dialogue; the service side of the physician relations role; and the ability to share concerns and needs with the rep and have them facilitate a solution. This makes sense, as these are attributes that can simplify their day-to-day work.

Physicians in our survey also value information on new physicians, which scored a 3.76 out of 5. There was no variation for primary care or specialists—they were in the same camp on this one.

This score was followed closely by helpfulness in sharing information about new programs at 3.72. As we see fewer primary care physicians (PCP) at the hospital, they are looking for easy methods to keep up with service offerings at their main hospital. This was evident in our scores, as the PCPs scored this at 3.81 and specialists gave it a 3.5.

In the survey group, another area that physicians scored in the high 3s was support with marketing their practice. Specialists are anxious to let referring physicians know about their practices. Many find the physician relations program to be a key way to inform others about their services—to market their practice. Perhaps not surprising, specialists scored much higher (specialists = 4.0 vs. PCPs = 3.4)

Updates on continuing medical education (CME) scored near the bottom. Physicians in our survey likely have access to the full array of CME offerings, so this is perceived to be less important to learn about in a face-to-face meeting.

The low score in this question was the rep's ability to bring internal leaders out to meet with them. Both primary care and specialists scored this low with the specialist score just a little higher at 3.1 vs. a 2.9 for the primary care group. We explored any difference in age and found none.

Respondents rated seven out of the 10 items above a 3.5 in terms of helpfulness, suggesting that the bulk of services provided by physician relations representatives are viewed positively and valued by physicians.

For everyone in the market who envisioned that a physician relations representative could assume the role as a link and a resource for physicians, this is great news. The role has officially moved from delivery of doughnuts and finding what is broken, to that of dialogue, a voice for leadership, and an effective conduit for concerns.

Resource Role

Practices are working harder and making less—that is not unique to them, but it has caused physicians to be even more careful about maximizing their efficiency. For most PCPs and more and more specialists, gone are the days of stopping into the doctor's lounge for a cup of coffee and conversation. The desire—and need—to see more patients has cost them in networking with their peers, informal updates on hospital changes, and partaking in educational offerings like grand rounds, tumor board, and medical staff meetings.

Informal ways to keep in touch are being replaced by e-mail and print updates, but those too require time. They also fall short in some of the communication nuances we get with personal connectivity. Misinformation, partial information, or information that has a "tone" has complicated the communication flow. Sometimes we are left feeling uncertain. The good physician relations rep can offer targeted information, customized to the physician's specific needs in a timely manner. The potential for this type of resource is significant. The obligation is to be a resource.

The following are attributes of needs-based dialogue:

- Preparation

- Good questions that surface the physician's topic of interest

- Ability to dialogue at a meaningful level

- Strong knowledge

- Connection to the right level of leadership for the right needs

- Ability to understand issues, to gather solid details about the concerns, and to manage them in a consistent way

Listening

Most physician relations representatives are fabulous talkers—that adage about people who could talk to a tree and have it talk back is not far from the truth. Yet, as these scores make clear, listening is perceived to be much more important than the talking.

Unfortunately, many physician relations reps feel the time pressure to get in and out. Wanting to be certain they tell physicians about the services, many reps have fallen into a show up and throw up routine. They get five minutes to offer an update, and they talk about their topic of interest with little time or attention to the doctor's topic of interest. They end with a question about concerns or problems and check the visit off the list. In the long term, this approach does not have the desired impact.

ATTRIBUTES OF GREAT LISTENING

I've heard it said that good listening is a habit. Here are six elements that are key to being a great listener:

1. Listen for meaning and relevance—be available

2. Restate and then further explore the physician's concept

3. Summarize and ask questions

4. Keep eye contact and jot down brief notes to retain content

5. Avoid distractions, including "what will I say next ..." dialogue in your head

6. Position yourself comfortably to engage and tune out other noise

---

Dialogue is earned through listening. It's interactive and often spontaneous conversation between the doctor and the representative. The doctors in this survey clearly told us they are interested in someone who can listen to their needs and who has the ear of leadership. Best practice programs are working hard to have their reps pre-plan approaches that offer an agenda, but then ask the physician if that agenda is of interest. They are prepared to ask a variety of questions and give the physician floor time. They have the right knowledge to respond after they listen to the physician's commentary.

GETTING THE LEADER'S BUY-IN

- No whining—provide facts that are actionable

- Be succinct

- Be prepared

- Include physician expectations

- Stage your learnings—let the leader know how you represent the organization

- Use data

- Listen to their points of view; dialogue is relevant here also!

Physician relations as the communicator

Whether it is an opinion, a complaint, an idea, or a question, what the physicians in this survey value most is that the representative is able to carry their feedback to the right level of leadership within the organization. As a rep, assuming that you have the leader's ear, are you sharing this ability as part of your dialogue with the doctor? The representative has the obligation to share what they will do with the information gleaned and when and how the physician will receive a response. To be effective in this role, the representative needs good internal knowledge of how topics are managed within the organization. They also need internal credibility.

The Complete Guide to Physician Relationships

C-suite engagement in your physician relations strategy

Physician relations programs today are perfectly poised to show business development value. And, with this, you have a unique opportunity to demonstrate your worth to the C-suite. The impact you make rests with your ability to effectively tell your story and position your results.

Physician relations reps should ask themselves what techniques and messages they can use to engage the C-suite, as well as how they can contribute to C-suite priorities in growing the referral base. Start by thinking strategically and performing tactically. See the big picture and think like an executive. What should the hospital–physician strategy look like? Help drive some of this thinking, and then get the results—perform tactically. One of the best things about what physician reps do is having the ability to gather some really great market and competitive intelligence. This information can help organizational leaders make strategic decisions. Listen for objective, relevant detail and understand your facility to know what information will matter most.

In your reports, show numbers. Show activity in physician-to-physician introductions, educational programs, volume, and physician satisfaction—whatever data makes sense for your organization and objectives. And talk about "wins." Beyond the formal reporting, look for opportunities to discuss any work you've done that positively contributed to the operational, strategic, or clinical functions of the organization. Keep it objective, factual, and brief, but do share in the appropriate settings and when the time is right.

Physician reps should assist C-suite members in developing a visit schedule for a select group of physicians. Choose physicians that you believe would benefit from their visits. Maybe you would like your executives to visit physicians with the most referral potential but are difficult to please, or with key opinion leaders or high-volume splitters.

Engaging your executive team in your efforts can lead to deeper relationships with the physicians. Many experts believe that collaboration between healthcare organizations and physicians will be the only way to prosper going forward. Your C-suite knows this. You can be a valuable resource to them as they search for the right approach and mode—and results.

Managing Concerns

Although relationship building is not a fishing expedition to learn what the organization is doing wrong, within a trusted relationship, the physician will feel comfortable in sharing their concerns about the organization with the representative. Doctors appreciate that they can tell one person and be confident that their message will be appropriately managed.

In addition, having a representative go to the practice leverages the opportunity to learn of concerns before they grow into big problems. The ability to resolve concerns scored better than a four of five in terms of value. Key to this factor is the resolution component, which has long been a challenge for many representatives. A decade ago reps tried to take on all the issues and fix them, and the result was that internal departments resented the rep and ignored the importance of the issue,

The Complete Guide to Physician Relationships

thus removing value from the solution. Today, many reps effectively gather the details of the concern and collaborate with the internal stakeholders to find a solution. The engagement of the internal staff with the physician in understanding their perspective has resulted in a powerful approach to managing issues on behalf of the physician.

INSIDER'S VIEW

MUTUAL ACCOUNTABILITY

"At Baptist Health, our physician relations sales team focuses on problem resolution and strategic service lines as defined by our senior leadership," says Mark Lowman, vice president of strategic development at Baptist Health in Little Rock, AR. "Our goal is to enhance relationships with our referring physicians while gaining new business opportunities with non-referring physicians," he says. "Our team operates in a results-oriented structure with clearly defined outcomes utilizing data to measure results. Each physician relations representative's outcomes are reviewed and reported to the CEO and senior management on a quarterly basis. The ability of the individual team members to interact directly with senior management across the organization has resulted in a feeling of mutual accountability by both executives and the reps."

Issue resolution cannot be addressed without a little commentary about the half-hearted approach that some internal staff have to responding to physician needs. Hospitals across the country have created huge systems and potent accountability roles to manage patient complaints. Most leaders would be appalled if they heard that one of their managers blew off a patient complaint. Yet very good organizations ignore or downplay physician complaints. I don't really understand it. It's not the doctor who complains about the lack of orange juice in the doctor's lounge that concerns me; it is the one who can share specific details about records not being sent or scheduling issues that are chronic problems. Assuming the physician complaint has actionable detail, and assuming they are a vital part of the organization's success, why don't we take the doctor's concern as seriously as we do the patient's?

The rep's obligation in managing concerns

Empathy is the key here. Listen carefully to the issue, and work hard to understand perception, personality, and level of expectation. Don't let your frustration with internal stakeholders influence you to sympathize against the organization. We've all been there—perhaps it is a repeat issue or the individual is a challenge. Having so many conversations about the things the organization is not doing right can push the rep into an adversarial position with his or her organization. The middle ground is the best place. Advocate for the doctor and the organization. Just think of the saying, "We know our own dirty laundry best."

Capture detail beyond emotion. When a physician shares a concern, gather details for the internal team that help them retrace their steps and problem solve. Use the who, what, when, where, why approach to provide facts to the internal stakeholders.

Respond quickly. A quick response may or may not come with a solution. It's about saying, "We heard you." Set a standard to make certain that the physician hears back within 48 hours or less with a message that says the concern is important. If there is a solution, provide it. If not, describe the actions in place to identify and solve the issue.

Department leaders are part of this. Whether the rep or the department head responds to the doctor is a matter of organizational preference. Personally, I believe there are times when it is very good for the internal stakeholders to have this conversation with the physician. It makes the issue more "real" for them; it adds a level of value for the physician to know the rep can make this happen. It also paints a picture of many individuals working to enhance the doctor's experience.

Reports are mandatory. Reporting key issues, their frequency, and the trends is essential. Leaders need to know that 70% of the surgeons targeted for more referrals are frustrated with our block schedule. The report should detail the top issues and include the responsiveness of departments, if that is an issue. This step moves us away from anecdotal stories that can be more subjective and more difficult to use to drive change.

Listening when they vent

Sometimes the conversation with the physician turns into a complaint session or a blow-off-steam opportunity for them—at the rep. Anyone who has been involved appreciates that what starts as a civilized conversation soon escalates into a grandiose event. It's clearly not the rep who is deserving of this; yet management of the issue and the conversation falls to them. When this occurs, it is important to listen to nuances, determine whether it is an isolated event, and, most importantly, uncover what the physician would have the representative do. It's fair to ask, "Dr. Smith, what would you have me do with this information?" and then give options. Example follow-up questions include, "would you like me to share this with our CMO, or the CEO?" or "is there additional data that I can gather for you?" Offering choices is good. The key elements are listening and offering to respond.

There is a limit to how many times the representative needs to be a part of this conversation. Assume this to be the rare interaction, not the norm. Frustration can reveal itself in many different ways—some get mad, some get even, and some just go away. Again, proactive communication in the practice creates the opportunity to probe more deeply and get attention to needs more quickly.

Helping Them Grow Their Practice

Growing the primary care practice

In our survey, the specialists rated this as more important than the primary care respondents by a score of 4.0 to 3.4. Is it because many PCPs are joining practices that are "too full," so practice building is a nonissue? Or perhaps they're employed with no personal financial incentive to be busier? With the shortage of primary care in many markets, they may see the challenge quite differently.

Yet, for the PCP, the representative can still play a key role in assimilating them into the medical community. The ability to introduce the primary care doctor to like-minded specialists is a real benefit. In addition, connections to educational offerings, streamlined service tools, an electronic medical record, or a portal are all value-added offerings that a physician relations rep can bring to the primary care practice.

PRACTICE MARKETING

If you are in a position to support practice marketing, Ann Maloley with Barlow/McCarthy offers these quick tips to get started:

- Understand the brand position

- Do your homework: understand current communication methods and the effectiveness

- Ask about access and service for patients and for referring physicians

- Analyze the opportunity

- Talk to the doctors

In the event that the primary care practice does need marketing help to find the right audience for practice growth, there are opportunities for support as well. The representative can support the practice by connecting them with the right talent to either purchase marketing support (for private practice) or align practice marketing staff (for employed practices). Again, the role is to be a proactive listener, anticipate needs, and ensure the right talent is in place to meet their needs.

We asked a question on the survey to learn more about what specialists perceive to be the best way to inform others about their clinical capabilities and expertise. This data slice is only meant to provide better understanding about how specialists want to be promoted (see Figure 10.2).

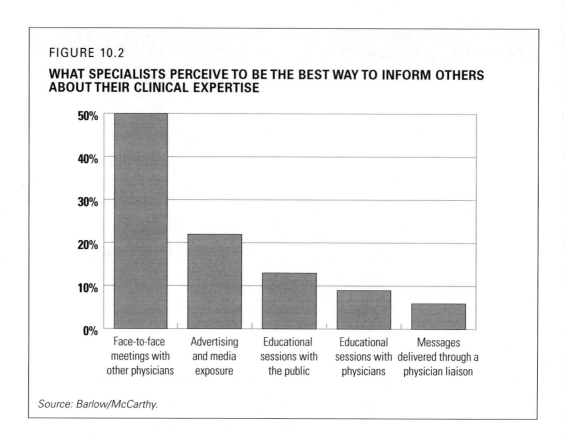

FIGURE 10.2

WHAT SPECIALISTS PERCEIVE TO BE THE BEST WAY TO INFORM OTHERS ABOUT THEIR CLINICAL EXPERTISE

Source: Barlow/McCarthy.

Even though the sample size is relatively small, we found specialists believe that face-to-face meetings with other physicians are the best way to communicate their expertise, according to 50% out of respondents. Another 22% of responding specialists are very interested in advertising and media exposure as a means to inform others about their expertise. Educational activities and programs with both the public (13%) and other physicians (9%) were viewed as less effective, and only 6% felt that the physician liaison was the best way to let other doctors know about their expertise.

The Complete Guide to Physician Relationships

Getting the word out

Many physicians still believe that promotion drives business. For example, the survey audience of specialists who responded still believe that advertising and media exposure is the best tool to inform the public about their expertise. The best way to measure this is by determining referral drivers. A 2008 Robert Wood Johnson survey concluded that 68.5% of specialist referrals are from a PCP. Other areas of referral are from friends (19.9%), from another physician (18%), through a health plan (10.5%), from the Internet (6.8%), and just 4.8% are other media. That is a striking disconnect, with 86.5% coming from another doctor and less than 12% from more consumer-oriented sources. Market awareness is important, and the role of consumerism cannot to be ignored. This finding shows why the doctors tend to be unhappy with the organization's focus on mass media. :their primary tool for driving image and awareness.

Inform and involve

Numbers speak to physicians. If you have a physician who is set on wanting media, the rep (and, sometimes, the marketing leader) can have a conversation about objectives, messages, and realistic tools. They will never change their opinion because someone says so, but they will consider data, case study examples, and an alternative process.

Obviously, there are legal considerations as well. The organization can position a hospital service but cannot provide the resources in any way that offers direct benefit to the practice if they're not employed. Be sure to seek advice from your legal counsel first, and then talk about marketing strategies with physicians. But don't use the legal defense and then back away.

Physician relations can work with members of the medical staff at every level to proactively offer information about what drives referrals and what we know consumers expect from doctors. Develop the platform from this approach—we want to collaborate, and we want to do it in the way that is best for your practice growth. Be proactive with informing and involving the doctors to manage some of the tension that is fueled by a belief that is not grounded in best practices.

Leveraging Education

Many organizations offer community education to showcase their doctors and their programs. This can take the form of face-to-face events, radio spots on health topics, Web videos, or other social media tools. Community education programs did not receive great ratings by the specialists, yet many organizations have anecdotally shared stories of success. Again, one must ask whether it's the approach or the lack of follow through to measure and then inform the masses that led to poor ratings. Even though these programs are likely have a few losers in the mix, many can be very successful in raising awareness. The next time you consider this approach, pre-plan for the metrics to determine success. Give the measurement detail to your physician relations team, and let them spread the word. We often get caught up in talking about issues and clinical happenings, but sometimes a little message about sharing the power of education is a nice proactive way to start or end a conversation with the doctor.

On-boarding

Many best practice organizations are now building practice support into the on-boarding plan for any new members of the medical staff. There is an opportunity to ensure that the strategy is not just limited to the employed doctors but open to all members of the medical staff. Specialists are anxious to practice medicine, and for some, this means introducing a new subspecialty that previously did not exist. For others, it may mean being the new person in a specialty area where another doctor or group has dominated for a long time. The survey validated that doctors refer to people they know, and survey respondents indicated that there is a role for physician relations in helping them get acquainted. Allison McCarthy and Ann Maloley offer the following on-boarding suggestions for what to put in place when integrating a newly recruited physician:

- Centrally managed process through a formal infrastructure of a multidisciplinary team with accountabilities

- Clear understanding of expectations—both the physician's and the hospital's

- Customized action plan by specialty, practice tenure, practice setting, and specific interests and needs

- Stakeholder introductions—administration, clinical, community

- Integration into the business aspects of the medical staff

- Detailed orientations to the hospital, practice, and community

- Integration needs for the family to get them personally oriented to the community

- Marketing and practice development discussions

- Post–on-boarding assessment to learn what you might have missed, three months later

- A tool that tracks turnover and the reasons why physicians leave

- Ongoing support and attention to their practice development and hospital engagement

Practice visits

In Chapter 9, we explored the need to make meetings with physician practices about more than a drive-through day. The representative needs to consider which practices are the right fit for meeting with the new specialist. The obligation is to be strategic and effective, rather than simply trying to check it off the list.

The Complete Guide to Physician Relationships

LIAISON'S ROLE IN PRACTICE DEVELOPMENT

"One of the biggest mistakes any hospital or health system can make is to invest a significant portion of their budget recruiting a physician and then spend nothing on helping the physician establish the practice and integrate into the medical staff and the community," says Pat Ball, senior vice president of strategic development and public affairs of LHP Hospital Group, Inc.

"Our company believes that one of the best strategies we have in our Physician Development program is the physician liaison component. In the case of practice development support, the physician liaison becomes the internal consultant to advise and direct the new physician as he or she is starting out. And with the seasoned physician, the liaison becomes the advocate or conduit for communication with other physicians or the administration. In both cases, the new or experienced physician will follow the lead of the liaison, as long as they perceive the activities to be of value and generate results."

Specialists want this service, so the rep has the opportunity to be more prescriptive in laying out his or her role and the role of the new specialist. Take charge, and drive the bus. As a marketing expert, the rep is the best person to define any pre-work, the agenda for the day, and intended follow-up. Let the physician know the plan by putting it in an e-mail or note. Own the obligation to follow up. In turn, the new specialist owns the obligation to track the referral impact. Ask for that metric—that's tracking you deserve.

Continue to connect

Knowing doctors like to have the representative introduce and support their practice development raises the questions of how much, with who, and how often. I have heard some reps say, "This could be my full-time job." Although the physicians like it and feel that it is a valuable service, there is a dose of reality in making this work for the representative.

Leading organizations in physician relations have assisted the rep by offering guidelines for both number and frequency of visits. Organizations are well served by formalizing the representative's role in creating connections for practice growth. A playbook for the physician that details other ways to practice build is an excellent value-added tool from the hospital. The playbook can call out the need for follow-up and many of the connection points discussed in the peer-to-peer chapters. It can also suggest other connection points within your organization—meetings, CME, or similar venues. Some organizations encourage members to participate in the physician newsletter or community events. It is important to encourage ongoing connections and to offer enough practical advice so that the doctor and/or practice will not be disappointed. The rep has an obligation to listen to the referring physician and to continue to match them with colleagues and/or services of interest.

What's Happening at the Hospital?

There are new challenges today that are a result of changes in communication patterns. Back in the day, there was less information to share, timeliness was less of an issue, and the methods were less intense. Because more work was done at the hospital, there was also more of an obligation to engage physicians. Those days are gone—there is no more catching up on hospital happenings at a medical staff meeting or poster in the doctors' lounge. Often, hospitals feel more inclined to have the doctors know about them than the doctors do about hearing. The survey score of 3.58 is likely an indication of the representative's need to be a good filter who shares only relevant detail. It is important to recognize that there is such thing as too much of a good thing.

Successful reps are doing this with dialogue—a conversation to stage what the physician wants to learn more about and then sharing updates. This is a very effective method.

The other method is to discern who in the practice needs which level of information. It is important to direct the message to the right audience. For example, the right message for the doctor is that the organization has a new hand surgeon who joined the staff last month. The right message for the referral coordinator is that the hand surgeon has a new phone line. The right message for the office coordinator is that the hand surgeon accepts the same insurance as their practice. This type of conversation does not fall into place unless the representative has clearly thought about it. As we continue to elevate the value of the rep's role for the physician, the content for dialogue needs to be relevant.

New doctor updates

Physicians always appreciate knowing about their peers—who is new on the staff, what is their experience, who have they joined, any special background, and any limitations. This detail can be provided on a card or flyer. The rep's role is more about connecting the type of patient within the practice and creating dialogue about potential. Remember that "tell and sell" is dead; the representative has the opportunity to learn more about real potential and to make certain they are not stepping on toes of existing referral sources by using dialogue to discuss the new physician.

Clinical news

The changing pace of technology and improvements in quality and safety are important messages to share with physicians—especially for those physicians who rely on hospitalists or who are specialists and rarely pay attention to hospital happenings outside of their specialized niche area. This is an important way to update those physicians who refer patients to the facility. Again, the representative needs to determine what is important, who is the right person to hear the detail within the practice, and how can it be shared in a way that engages the doctor in meaningful conversation. If you don't need a conversation and it is a pure data dump, then respect the doctor's time—perhaps then this score for value will go from a B+ to an A for the next survey.

Politics and the inside scoop

Let's be honest: Talk is a billion-dollar industry outside of healthcare, and we are not immune. Some doctors really enjoy learning what's going on and find the representative their best internal source. But be careful here—conversation about happenings is great, but beyond that, it can get most representatives into a place that is very hard to get out of. Carefully frame the role to ensure that the physician feels informed and involved, without it becoming gossip. And it is always fair to ask, "Interesting that you should ask; what have you heard?" The best offered hospital updates in this category fall to details that were printed in a newsletter or shared at a medical staff meeting—and then repeated by the rep.

Business deals

Many of the physicians do not see their representative as a conduit for business strategy. The assumption is that this is market specific. Some reps are asked to soften the market and introduce business options to interested practices. Those programs that have implemented this are seeing good success, so the trend may grow. Likely, the proportion of those interested will never be as large as a number of practices have already made changes or decided they are not interested in a business relationship with the hospital. Although the score was low, those that are interested seem to very much appreciate that the liaison is informed and offers a connection.

Creating links with leadership

The lowest scorer in terms of value from the rep is the need to bring leaders to the practice. Frankly, I was bummed about this. More and more organizations have leaders who are willing to join their reps in the practice, and it seems like an excellent way to connect and let the two parties engage. Do the doctors just not care? Have the leaders failed to engage in dialogue? Was there another agenda here that was not productive? In any regard, moving forward, the representative has an obligation to do a better job of determining when this strategy is in play. These visits need to be orchestrated so the discussion has good value for both parties. Using the "what can we do for you?" question is clearly not the answer.

If as a representative you have been actively engaged in leadership meetings with the practices, query the practices to learn of their perceived value. Ask them, on a 1 to 5 scale, if 5 is excellent, how they would score the value of having a hospital leader come to your practice for a conversation with you. Then ask one more question: If they were to come, which of these topics are of most interest? Give them three choices. The obligation here is to learn whether it is the idea or the execution that is pulling the score down. In some markets, it could just be personalities.

Summary

Many practices now rely on the physician relations representative to be a communications liaison. The role is appreciated when it is needs-based and perceived to have a direct line to leadership. The ease of having a single person for sharing concerns is also very valued. The challenge for every representative is to continue to add this value for the practice and to ensure that the end result is something of value within the organization. Consultative relationship sales enable the representative to focus on the physicians needs and customize solutions based on the organization's product offerings.

> *"The elevator to success is out of order. You'll have to use the stairs …*
> *one step at a time."*
> —Joe Girard

Many great representatives have already paved the way; the challenge is that what works today will likely not be effective tomorrow. Ongoing surveys, like this one, done locally, can be merged with good field intelligence and assessments of the field impact to create the right future model—before it's required.

Physician Relations Attributes That Matter

The physicians who responded to our survey count on physician relations representatives to prioritize their need—65% stated that the most important attribute of the representative is knowing what is most important to their practice's success (see Figure 11.1).

Having influence and a direct connection with the CEO and C-suite are also important attributes, according to 49% of physicians. Being connected to the leaders of the organization was more important for the specialists than the primary care respondents.

In addition, 49% of survey respondents said it is important that the representative be able to influence hospital decisions. The overall sentiment of the physicians surveyed indicates a desire for support to streamline their requests and the process for working with the hospital.

Physicians rely heavily on their staff—40% of respondents cited the ability of reps to build relationships with staff as important. And having a clinical background was the least important attribute, as noted by 19% of survey respondents.

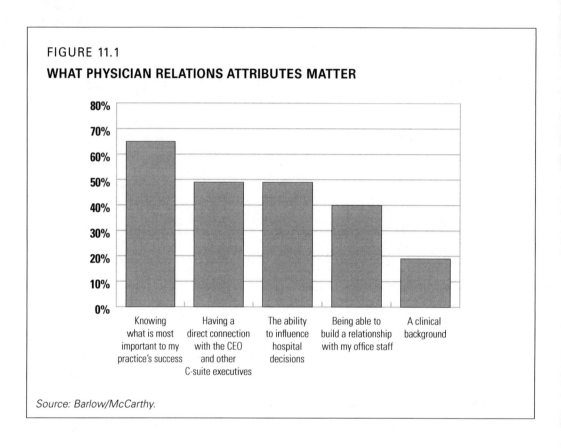

FIGURE 11.1

WHAT PHYSICIAN RELATIONS ATTRIBUTES MATTER

Source: Barlow/McCarthy.

The Relationship Is About Physicians

Based on this survey, there is no doubt that physicians desire to have a representative who is able to relate to their needs. They want someone who can articulate what their needs are and deliver on them. Physicians understand that the organization is motivated to earn referrals—they get it. But the fact that 65% of physicians noted the relationship is about understanding the practice reveals that there is a need for a high-level person to engage physicians in a conversation about

The Complete Guide to Physician Relationships

what matters to them. This seems to be the gateway for any type of relationship to flourish.

To pave the way to understanding individual practices and the dynamics within them, it's important to have a general sense, first, of how practices function. One thing we know for sure: The practice environment is changing, and physicians are feeling the pressure. Their practice costs are rising, and their reimbursements are declining. They have less time to spend with each patient and, at the same time, patients are demanding more time. And let's not forget about the competition that physicians are dealing with every day as they work to capture the most desirable patients, while being challenged by other practices and healthcare organizations competing for that same business.

Physician reps should keep these and other factors in mind as they begin to engage with practices to demonstrate that they understand what's important to the practice's success.

Understanding the life within a practice

How much of the representative's orientation is about understanding the practice? Probably not much. The survey findings are a reminder of the need to make sure that representatives understand the roles within the practice, the office dynamics and hierarchy, and what is managed by whom—including decisions that are left to the individual implementer. It is also helpful to have a general sense of the business process within practices and the typical challenges of running a practice in today's environment. Most practices run lean, so individuals may wear many hats. Take the time to understand the workings of those key practices as the doctor is expecting it.

The opportunity to shadow may be an option for the representative as well. If this is done, make certain that nuances are detailed so others on your team can benefit from this experience. The following are some guidelines:

- It is a great time to determine whether there are pet peeves—especially as it relates to reps and their office time.

- Make certain that there is good planning with quality questions so it proves worthwhile for all involved.

- It's not just about learning what happens; it is an inside look at relationships within the practice and understanding roles.

- Observe what gets attention from the doctors and what does not.

- Get a sense of the mood of the clinic to understand attitudes and expectations.

If shadowing is not an option, take advantage of any office manager meetings to gain understanding of their environment. It can be meetings in their practice or educational events with a large group. Asking the right questions over a period of time can increase awareness of the practice pace, challenges, expectations, and desired approach. For example, in meetings with the office manager in the practice ask, "Is there a time of year that your practice does more business planning?" Or at your office managers' luncheon, ask on a comment card, "What is the best time for other physicians to connect with physicians in your practice?"

It is about putting together a profile of what makes the practice tick. The best relationships are those that are grounded in a sensitivity to and respect for unwritten rules. And remember, every practice is different. Do not assume that learnings from one shadowing experience will provide a model for every practice—it's just a start.

Personal Development for This Role

Even if today's successful physician relations representative has worked to advance his or her skills, the nuances of this relationship go beyond the right look or the ability to articulate the service details for the hospital. The doctors said they want the representative to understand their needs. That means having the right conversations at the right level. Good conversations at this level rarely happen without some preparation and a lot of work at skill development.

There are many types of representatives who visit the practice every day. Consider how you can stand out and earn the right level of positioning. For instance:

1. Actions speak louder than works. If relationship counts first, then work to earn that relationship.

2. Manage your materials. As you observe other reps, you will notice that they feel the need for a leave-behind every time. To differentiate, your leave-behind might be a summary of actions you will provide as a result of the conversation.

3. If you are not acting like another sales rep, then you have the opportunity to be positioned differently. Move out of vendor row in the reception area so you are not associated as one of them. Add value, and you will be received differently.

4. Recognize every member of the practice with messages that are relevant to their work needs.

5. Always make sure that the timing you have selected is good for them. Courtesy is a great relationship builder.

6. Ask for one-to-one dialogue with the doctor, unless you are bringing another specialist or stakeholder to present. This sets the stage for a discussion versus a presentation—and it gives the rep the chance to learn about needs of those doctors beyond the one who frequently speaks at meetings.

INSIDER'S VIEW

ASKING THE RIGHT QUESTIONS

Physicians want to know they've been heard, says Susan Boydell, director of business growth strategy at Texas Health Resources. Identifying a physician's needs and expectations is the starting point. Begin by asking the right questions, listening to their answers, and then asking more questions. There is a gem in each of those conversations. Acting on what you learn is one of the most powerful approaches to ensuring a long-term meaningful relationship.

The Complete Guide to Physician Relationships

Less talk, more good questions

It has been said that nothing can build rapport like a great question. It is the single most essential attribute for relationship building with physicians and their practices. It immediately moves the representative from someone who is pushing a product or telling the practice about how great they are into a different space. When you ask the right question, the physician's mind shifts to answer it. When the question is about them and their needs, you are in the right space to engage, learn more, and begin to understand how they make decisions.

Not all questions are good ones, however. There are two questions that I really don't like. The first is, "How's it going?" This question really does nothing to engage the physician and feels like a filler for empty space. The other one may not feel as obvious at first. It is, "What can we do for you?" At a glance, it feels very open and portrays willingness. However, if I am the physician, you put all of the onus on me—it requires the doctor to inventory their needs and then reply. More often than not, what the representative will learn is a top-of-mind problem. It may or may not be a difference maker for them, and it is almost certainly not strategically linked to relationship building.

A better approach to asking questions is to demonstrate an understanding of physician needs and that of their practice.

The following are attributes of great questions. They should:

- Create an immediate picture in my mind.

- Be succinct and well phrased.

- Be planned and have a reason, which could be information, attitude, rapport building, or positioning to introduce a service benefit. Different reasons need different types of questions.

- Point in the direction of another question or dialogue on a topic you know to be of interest to the doctor.

- Start with a "what" or "how" or a "tell me more" word to solicit more than just a yes or no reply. Sometimes yes/no are needed, but as rapport is built, try to engage more dialogue through open-ended questions.

Consider these as examples: How are referral decisions made within your practice? What's most important to you in a joint replacement program? What percentage of your practice is over the age of 55? How would you like me to share relevant news about our new surgeons?

Skills to message this

The representative's goal is to learn more about the practice and their needs, and good questions are a great tool. But even the best questions are not enough to earn great rapport—it takes the total package. Sometimes it is helpful to start with what does not work and then work back to define the right approach for your relationship with the practice.

What do practices tell us they dislike about reps?

- It's that there is an "all about me" attitude. Many reps will come into the practice and proceed to offer a litany of every service they are promoting without taking the time to learn about needs.

- Dropping by without regard for their patient schedule. Drop-bys can work, but it's important to gauge the activity in the clinic to know whether the time is right to ask to see the physician.

- Asking for time with the doctor without a good plan and clear objective. This also generally goes down the path of too much dumping the bucket and too little needs-based dialogue. To the physicians and staff, this is seen as wasting their time.

- Disingenuous behavior will make the office staff nuts! For example, if the rep asks for five minutes to discuss a survey result and then does a bait and switch using the time to talk about their product, it may be their last visit. Members of the practice talk, so it is really important to do what you say you will and do it in the time requested.

Finding your style

Seasoned representatives have honed their style and approach for working with practices. Some use enthusiasm and high energy, whereas others may be warm and relaxed or have a quiet, confident approach. As you observe seasoned field colleagues, you'll see them move into their zone in a consistent and disciplined way.

Just make sure your style is congruent with the style of your audience. In a low-key practice, over-the-top energy is likely to go over like a lead balloon.

Taking the DISC assessment profile for sales, which stands for dominance, influence, steadiness, and compliance, is a great way to learn your personal style. It also highlights those attributes that you need to address to be successful in earning rapport with others. Whether it is a profile, a 360 interview tool, input from teammates, or assessment from leaders, the representative needs to really pay attention to style and approach. Few jobs require as much personal assessment as those that are grounded in relationships. Successful representatives are constantly looking for new ways to connect and create rapport—it's a skill that takes effort.

What's In It for Me?

The surveyed physicians called out the value of the representative who knows what is important to the practice. Beyond asking questions and great listening, another way for the representative to demonstrate their understanding is by reflecting on what the doctor shared in previous meetings. For example, if the doctor shared a concern about wait times in the emergency room and the rep is trying to showcase the department on the next visit, they should bring detail about the actual wait times. If it is a trouble spot, the follow-up needs to include actions and timeline for resolution. The ability to provide good follow-up visibly demonstrates that the representative understands the practice needs and that he or she is an advocate for the doctor.

<table>
<tr><td rowspan="2">INSIDER'S VIEW</td><td>

TWO-WAY COMMUNICATION IS VITAL

Establishing mechanisms for continuous two-way communication with our regional clinicians is the foundation for our program. We base our internal efforts on feedback from the regional physicians. For example, both our regional clinician service center (physician consultations) and our hospital admissions center were developed as a result of feedback from community physicians throughout the four-state area.

—*Darlene Corkrum, senior vice president, marketing and chief marketing officer, and Catherine Kennebeck, administrative director, strategic markets at Virginia Mason Medical Center*

</td></tr>
</table>

The leader's ear

Physicians expect that the feedback provided to the representative will reach the right level of leadership. This obviously includes complaints, but that's not all. When a good relationship with the practice is developed, representatives get a good sense of the practice's clinical and business needs and expectations. And because many physicians do not feel close enough to members of the leadership to pick up the phone, and they may not be at the hospital that often, these messages don't get communicated. In these cases, they value the role that the representative can play in sharing their perspectives.

Demonstrate this

The representative needs to position his or her willingness to be a conduit for information in face-to-face meetings with the doctor. Recognize that others may have promised action in the past. If it did not happen, it will take a little proof for the physician to have confidence and share freely. As part of the dialogue, the rep needs to let the doctor know about his or her involvement with the leaders. For example, "I learned something in my meeting with Ms. CEO last week that I wanted to make sure to share with you."

Connect the dots

The physician may need some help understanding the role the representative plays within the organization, and the influence that role may have in driving infrastructure and communication needs and business development strategy. When necessary, articulate the ways you interface with leadership. Do you have regular meetings with them? Do you interface with them in internal meetings where you have the opportunity to formal share information from the field? Show how the information they share will get back to leadership.

Wise use of confidential details

It is a fine line to walk between confidante and "chief messenger." Sometimes it is worth an extra question just to make sure that you clearly understand what was meant to be shared and what was just conversation. If in doubt, simply ask, "Is this detail something you'd like me to share with your name on it, anonymously, or not at all?" Better to be safe than sorry on this one.

Not a fishing expedition

There are times when the internal stakeholders may like to turn this role around. Just as the doctors like the reps' direct connection to leadership, the leaders like that the rep is able to gather learnings from the doctor. Both parties understand the engagement here; just make certain that the desire to gather field intelligence does not leave the doctor feeling exposed. The representative needs to have long-term credibility with the practice. It is never earned if they believe the hospital sent an individual just to gather "scoop" about them.

Representatives need to be coached to understand the nuances of this. If the representative does not have great intuition and finesse, this will be a struggle. Back to the number one expectation again: It is important to the doctor that the representative understands their success.

Not just conversation for the sake of conversation

The doctors in our survey clearly told us that they expect the representative to be able to speak up for their needs at the hospital level. With 49% stating that it is important for the representative to be in a position to influence hospital decisions, the role of advocate for the practice is really carved out. How are representatives actively influencing business decisions? Consider creating a template that measures your influence and helps you track where you can be more influential (see box "Business Decisions Influence").

BUSINESS DECISIONS INFLUENCE			
	Yes, influencing now	Not influencing currently, but potential area	Not a fit— reason
• Outreach education			
• Referral communication protocols			
• Communication about ACO plans			
• Patient scheduling			

A voice

Time, energy, and the organization's business process may all be areas that interfere with the doctors' feeling that they can impact change. Before the representative role was fully developed, the doctor either had to seek out a leader or just ignore the issue. Although some organizations still have a strong, cohesive medical staff, in many locations, there is a distance and lack of synergy because of the challenges stated earlier. As a result, the doctors are more reliant on individual voices that can be melded into themes and influence decisions through the rep. The representative can give the doctor a voice.

Gaining traction internally

The doctors indicated that they expect the representative to have influence with senior leadership. They expect their messages about business-related needs to be communicated to leadership effectively. It begs these questions:

- If you are a representative, do you have the right level of rapport with senior leaders?

- If you are a leader, do you have a representative that can earn this rapport with doctors and leaders?

- Is there a process in place to filter and evaluate feedback that is gathered in the field?

- Does the leadership team understand the priorities at the practice level?

- Do the leaders take the feedback from the field to heart? Do they respond quickly and assure the physician that their method of connecting with the rep is the right approach?

The physician relations team is in a great position to elevate feedback from the field to where leaders will find it valuable for business strategy. Take on this responsibility, and build a process that is suitable to the culture of the organization and of the leadership team.

Managing Internal Perception

It is the obligation of the representative to be the consummate communicator from the field. This is not effective if it is done one message at a time or if it is only fielding a regular stream of complaints. And it does not matter how compelling the story is if it follows three or four similar stories that were delivered in the same week. It is not about whether this is right or wrong; it is just reality. The most effective method to earn the ear of leadership is to use a combination of numbers and stories.

Use data to influence decisions

The ability to roll up concerns and put patterns to them will enhance the impact. For example, 72% of primary care physicians visited this quarter indicated that they were unable to schedule a MRI within three days. This type of communication moves leaders to action because it shows a consistent problem in an area that they desire to grow.

Data is also impactful when the representative desires to demonstrate the level of internal responsiveness. In this case, it might be that last month, 12 scheduling concerns were shared with radiology. A response to the concern was generated within our desired time of 48 hours only 30% of the time.

When this type of data is combined with one of "those stories" that makes the patient experience real for leaders, the representative gains the level of traction that the physicians expect.

Know what can't be influenced

Although the physician—and the rep—would love more authority, it's not an all-inclusive path to control. And the ultimate no-no is to promise what you are not able to deliver. It is important to frame the role for the doctors so they understand that although the representative is absolutely their advocate and a great conduit for their needs, there is no guarantee. Physicians understand this but will still try for more—that is human nature. The seasoned representative will be able to clearly articulate, "Here's what I can do, here's what I can't, and here's why. And if I should do this, here's what I believe will be the outcome that benefits you—and that benefits my organization." And it's important to have this conversation when the physician makes a request, not after the fact. Doing so later makes it look like an excuse, and this chips away at your credibility.

Office staff inclusive

Forty percent of the physicians say the importance of the representative's ability to build a relationship with their office staff is key. Many doctors rely on their staff to communicate their needs to the representative. This is especially true when the need is about access or efficiency, as those are topics of most importance to staff. Although some practices may have a revolving chair at the front desk, many practices have had staff members in place for a long time. They run the mechanics of the practice. And they have a significant role in directing referrals, especially for all the outpatient diagnostics, testing, and follow-up care.

Defining the relationship with staff

The representative's work with office staff is complicated. The same staff that can be grueling gatekeepers are also essential sources for information about referral relationships. The balance is to understand their needs, just like you do for the doctor. Often the staff is much more interested in the day-to-day detail of getting referrals into a facility or scheduling an exam. It is important to understand the role they play and then provide information—and value—to them.

The relationship with staff can not preclude a relationship with the doctor. It is not an either/or situation. Both have different needs; both need to be informed, to be listened to, and to feel that the organization values the relationship with them. However, the conversations are different. It is about the needs of the doctor, but it is also about the opportunity to engage in conversations about care delivery and referral needs. Although some would say that the staff makes all the referral decisions, experience says that the staff is given leverage to manage the referrals for most ancillary services almost exclusively. However, in the case of inpatient procedures, all it takes is a doctor to state, "I do not want referrals going to ACME General," and the best office staff relationship in the world will not save the referrals. Relationships need to be with both parties. The representative can work to support the efforts of each member of the practice.

Engage the office staff

Many programs have strong tools in place to work with their office staff. Education on their topics of interest is always popular. Some organizations do other events or facilitate ways to give the staff a chance to meet the people they interface with at the hospital. Consider what fits best for your program. Consider the time it takes away from the field and the cost. Once you consider the options, test your ideas with office staff in your market to ensure that they match their needs.

Clinical expertise

In this survey, 19% of the doctors felt that a clinical background was an important attribute for the representative. In the *Physician Relations Programs in Hospitals 2010: A SHSMD Benchmarking Study*, 23% of the respondents had a clinical background. Organizations across the country often ask about this. In both surveys, it seems to be of most value when there is a clinical service that is highly specialized, such as transplant or in specialty hospitals where referring physicians are commonly specialists referring to other specialists.

Nonclinical representatives need to have a solid background in the service offerings and a good understanding of the process that brings patients from the practice to that service. The ability to have a conversation about a service is also dependent on the representative understanding what differentiates the services. And, remember, if this is about meeting their needs, likely they get the clinical piece; more often than not the conversation will be related to access or service. If the conversation needs to be clinical, this presents a great opportunity to bring in a clinical counterpart from that service line to help support the sales effort.

Based on the survey, it seems to be more about good, caring communication and the ability to get the attention of leadership than it is about understanding clinical matters at a complex level.

Summary

Physician relations staff add value for the physicians by understanding their needs and acting as a conduit for communication to the hospital leaders. The expectation is that communication with the rep can help create a link as physicians spend less time in the hospital and yet wish to have their needs, ideas, and challenges shared with leadership. Perhaps this is another sign of the challenge doctors face with maximizing efficiency—they opt to have a conversation with the representative because it is easier.

The role of the physician representative is currently secure, but success in that role today does not ensure that it will be the same tomorrow. There is a constant need to test the market and to learn what adds value for the doctors, the practice, and the organization that is represented. But no matter how the environment evolves, speaking to physicians on their terms and supporting their needs will be central to any strategy. Good conversations are at the heart of this learning for the future.

Physician Relations' Voice

For everyone who is in physician relations as a leader or working in the field, I say, game on! The takeaway from this survey is that physician relations has evolved and plays a pivotal role in the communication that an organization has with its physicians. It is now about seizing what's working and enhancing it to meet the needs of the doctor, the practice, and the organization represented. It is also about living in today's climate, with one eye toward the future.

The focus of this chapter is to call out what's working and why, and then to detail those attributes that can differentiate programs and add value for their physicians. The face-to-face relationship sales approach has many advantages. For example:

- It's personal. With so many other message formats, this one is about people. It feels different, and it gives a sense of connection.

- It can be customized. Messages are not delivered with a one-size-fits-all approach. Just because you are an OB/GYN physician, you may not want to talk about gestational diabetes. The ability to ask good questions and create a conversation based on what the doctor wants to discuss is a positive.

- Only relevant topics earn floor time. Messages that are shared with the doctor and questions that are asked are planned but not forced—this ensures pertinent and interesting content. Physicians tell us that they are tired of too many messages from their facility of choice that are not relevant to their needs. This approach gives ample opportunity to ensure relevance.

It's clear that the desired model—to meet the needs of all parties—is not a pure sales model. Long-term relationships need more than updates and insights on products to provide the glue that keeps them strong. The model is also not just relationships; the relationship needs to have a purpose, be progressive, and move both parties toward a beneficial outcome. The best model is sensitive to the needs of both parties and naturally has more of a consultative feel; it uses sales skills to earn the right level of relationship and to gain commitment. Clearly, this is a specialized role, and talent will need to be cultivated for ongoing success.

Expanding the Role

Historically, physician relations/liaisons were heavily reliant on practices making time to hear from reps. Now that everyone wants a few minutes with doctor, however, their time is even more limited. At the same time, the practice is feeling tremendous pressure to increase their volumes, so setting aside time for reps, of any type, has become very challenging.

Today, representatives are spending more time prospecting and getting meetings. I hear, "It's hard to get to the doctor, let alone have a meaningful conversation." There are longer cycles with more up front work with the office staff, and many are frustrated because they cannot "hit their numbers." It sounds like a car heading down a dead end street. Physicians have less time, so reps push harder. Doctors feel limited value—and sometimes resentment—from the "push" and the old "show up and throw up" method.

As this survey illustrates, doctors need a representative that understands and communicates their desires. This is hard to do with two minutes in a hallway. In the near term, the rep is able to count the visit as an outcome of the effort, and there may be times when results do follow. However, in the long run, this is not getting to the real value proposition. When the rep shifts from adding value to becoming "just another rep," it is a bad news situation for physician relations professionals.

Creating a change environment is complex, and a multitude of books have been written on the subject. But change doesn't need to be a total do-over with wholesale change to your model. Let's focus on four areas: data, differentiation, knowledge and integration. As you develop your long-term approach, consider where you are with this content. If there is need to improve, then create a plan for evolving your approach.

Gather Data, Use Data, Show Your Impact With Data

There are two essential uses of data for a solid physician relations effort:

1. To determine which doctors are right for the personal visit

2. To demonstrate the impact

Obviously they are related, but not all programs have both of the components working as they desire. Better research and use of data means that you understand:

- The types of data that are available and the perceived accuracy

- The way senior leadership looks at data and uses it in business decisions

- Scope of the effort to gather data and the go-to person to make it happen

Much of this element will be transparent to the doctor and the relationship. But the doctors told us they expect the representative to have the ear of the leadership. And what gets their attention? You guessed it: Data.

Business planning within physician relations

Many programs have excellent targeting strategies and have taken the time to evaluate which doctors are loyal and need to be retained and which ones offer the potential for more referrals. If you have not, the time is now, because having a defined group of physicians that you plan to visit stages everything else that you do.

Before you research which doctors to see, spend time determining the organization's expectations, and take an internal look at your program realities. This may include:

- Strategic direction established by leadership

  – Services that are designated for growth

- Their desire and then approach for stronger linkages with loyal doctors

- Market-driven payer and/or managed care realities

• Services that the organization wishes to expand

• Service and care delivery needs

• Market and climate

- Role of primary care physicians in the local market

- Physician employment in the market and how "locked in" they are

- Business relationships formed by the competition

- Distinctions between local, regional, or national referral base

- Physician perceptions of your organization

• Number of relations staff

In other words, before you launch an all-out data mining process, set a framework of knowing what you want from the data and what you will do with it once it's all gathered. Data can clearly tell the story, but only if you are clear about the type of story you want.

Using existing data specific to individual physicians is preferred, but work with what you have. Sometimes that means specialist-only data, data sorted by patient ZIP code, or the service line referral patterns. Look for trends in the data.

The goal is getting to a summary that details a defined group of physicians, by category, and that offers the right potential to meet the goals of your physician relations program. Targeting is tedious and can be a bit painful at times. It is also a step that I would never want to exclude.

Demonstrate impact

The "right data to measure results" is a limitless topic of conversation in referral development circles. Although some organizations have much better data for this than others, even if you purchase a perfect database, it will need attention. Successful programs use the data they have to show their effort is having an impact.

The starting point is, again, to understand what your organization values. A simple example, some leadership teams are focused on contribution margins, some want to see an up-tick in outpatient only, and others are interested in growth of the key service lines. Once you know what you could provide in this regard, create a sample report. Share the sample with your CEO, COO, CFO, and CMO, and let them select their preferred approach.

Next, make sure that what they value can be achieved. Often the vice president of business development or marketing, or a chief medical officer, may need to weigh in. If there are tremendous challenges with service delivery in a clinical area, putting more attention on them will only heighten the issue. The risk is that you may be pouring new referrals in the top of the funnel, only to have them run out the bottom. Perhaps in this case, time and resources should be spent in working first with those who are more loyal to create physician-driven solutions. Or pick another service for focus.

In a perfect world, the data would capture every admission by primary care doctor, through the specialist, and then into a clinic or hospital setting—but, without significant investment, this may not be feasible for you. Although you can become an internal advocate for better systems to capture referrals internally, don't wait for data to be perfect. Use what you have. Some organizations can measure regional referrals by changes in ZIP code volume. Others need to select 20 specialists that they are growing referrals through to measure inpatient volumes.

At the end of the day, future success and program recognition will come to those who do the research to determine the optimal targets and then consistently demonstrate the impact. Measure and report to show your value within the organization.

Listen to Differentiate

Because of the pace—in the practice and for the reps—an insidious shift has moved many away from relationship sales to detailing (pitching) in the practices. Now many will quickly point out that pharmaceutical sales have successfully detailed practices for decades, so why not replicate? The simple answer is that replicating that model offers nothing that differentiates your organization. The rep then becomes just one of many. Even when they see you, if you are telling them what you think they should be interested in learning, the results are mixed at best. And we rarely have products that are clearly defined, like they have in pharma.

The physician relations rep has the opportunity to be in a space that many pharma reps would envy, because the doctors in this survey *want* a representative who understands their practice. They see the representative as their link, which offers a host of opportunities.

Physician relations reps have a tremendous opportunity to create a very different level of relationship with the practice and the doctor—as long as they have the right knowledge. By creating a real needs-based dialogue, there is opportunity to understand the wishes of the physician and their practice and to position your organization's offerings. And well-defined questions play an important role. It is much easier to dump the bucket of information, but it is more fruitful to create the dialogue-based relationship we want.

Successful needs-based selling generally requires internal education about the way practices make referral decisions. It is amazing how many internal stakeholders think that if we just "tell them what we offer" the business will come flying in. In today's market, the business you desire is going to someone else. The only way to earn those referrals is to clearly differentiate your product and/or services in a consistent manner. Help your leaders understand this process, and then demonstrate how effective you can be. Be sure to call out that the services they ask you to sell must be ready for new business. Challenge any service and access issues that you see as a satisfaction barrier—if there are any—so that you don't lose credibility by selling something that won't provide a good experience for the referring physician, their patient, or both.

Please don't construe relationship and needs-based to mean that we are not selling, because that is far from my intended message. This is not asking what's wrong and filling a notebook with issues that we cannot fix; this is focused relationship selling. Doctors want to be involved and included in the areas that are relevant to them, so use a model that accomplishes that. Those who will be successful in the future will have the ability to learn about the physicians' needs and focusing on areas where the hospital has opportunity. There will be a consistent approach to positioning the attributes and gaining commitment.

Knowledge Is an Obligation

As a rep, if you want to be a resource, you need to be knowledgeable. This does not mean that you need to know everything about all the clinical offerings, but you do have to be a good student: gathering relevant information for the select doctors you will be visiting, refining your knowledge, asking good questions, knowing how the referral chain works, and preparing your benefit-oriented messages based on what you learn. It's about listening and sharing with the right level of leadership, and for most, it's not important to be a clinician. I believe it is important to understand clinical information so you can connect with them in their comfort zone.

Clinical staff have a wonderful understanding of their areas but will not always think about it from an outside-in point of view. It is your job to fully prepare to interview them, with that focus. It is wrong to assume that they will feed you all the information you need to connect from the physician's perspective and/or to grow referral relationships. Work hard to research the clinical expertise of your organization, the data that demonstrates this, and the best way to use this to connect with the prospective physician.

Internal Coordination, Collaboration, Integration

This category brings us to the fourth key area that emerged from the survey results. Perhaps I fell short in not asking a few more questions to learn what the doctors want from operations staff. Although it was not covered in the survey, it does need to be called out as an area of attention for the physician relations team.

Within health systems, there is a push for brand consistency. The brand that we share with our consumers needs to be visibly demonstrated in our actions with the medical staff. This means that we refine our messages and then consider how our messages match the delivery.

Individuals who are inside the care delivery system see the world from their perspective, which is mostly about patient care once a patient is admitted. They rarely consider how the referral was earned, how a seamless process for access made an impact, or how a lack of communication back to a doctor may impact the next referral. Assembly line thinking has everyone doing their job with no thought beyond it. The result is that even those organizations that have outstanding clinical teams find themselves losing ground to organizations that make themselves easier to use. This is one of those elements that physician relations will not solve; however, there is much work that can be done to create a more inclusive approach and to provide data that calls out practice needs and expectations.

Proactive positioning is key. When internal stakeholders are asked about the physician relationship, the ultimate goal is that they see it as a continuum that starts with external messages delivered by the sales team, with support of

The Complete Guide to Physician Relationships

marketing, and then a dependence on their internal efforts to deliver in a consistent manner. And, yes, this is so easy to say and so hard to accomplish. With so many involved, leadership needs to own and support this as it is about a culture of involvement and with each person doing their part.

Beyond integration with our clinical and patient centered services, the call center, the medical staff office, marketing, public relations, and planning are impacting relationships with the medical staff every day. Programs that take the first steps in collaboration will benefit from enhanced awareness of internal messaging that impacts physicians. Alignment of the brand message for consumers—and physicians—can clearly make your organization different in a cluttered market.

> The majority of physician relations managers noted that their staff are reasonably effective—garnering a 3.9 score on a 1 to 5 scale—at interfacing with service line leaders today.
>
> Source: *The Society for Healthcare Strategy & Market Development's 2010 Physician Relations Survey.*

Get introspective

Take a look at how far you have come with your program—a pat on the back is likely well deserved. Next, set a goal for your program. I recently spoke to a program leader who said, "I want us to be one of those programs that is called out when you look at best practices in the country." That is certainly an achievable goal with focused effort. Define your goal for the next year, and for three years down the road. Take the time to do an honest assessment of these four areas, and perhaps other needs within your program, and then create a plan. It has been said that if you really want change, the first step is to realize you have to change those systems that created the current culture. The pressure is on in our marketplace, so take the leap and create a model that can position you for success.

Own the collaboration

The premise of this book is understanding the doctors' expectations of communication with four key groups: physician relations, marketing, leadership, and peers. Physician relations has the opportunity to play a pivotal role in the communication link within these three groups. Marketing is interested in producing materials that are relevant and meaningful to the doctor. Physician relations staff can help communicate physician priorities and share the practice perspective. And you will know best what messages will resonate and how to shape them. Identify what other ways you can interface with marketing communications and the organization's marketing strategy to extend the brand and ensure message consistency.

Leadership is actively engaged in discussions with physicians about accountable care, quality drivers, and engagement strategies. Physician relations can be a conduit for sharing messages about the hospital patient experience and outcomes. This is the type of information our doctors want, and the rep can deliver it on behalf of leadership. Leaders are more broadly connected to the medical community, which can sometimes make it difficult to communicate the detail. Determine the information that the leaders want to hear from doctors that could be consistently gathered by physician relations. What are the specific messages that leadership would like to share with targeted physicians? Beyond just field intelligence, consider offering meaningful impressions related to new models of care delivery.

Physician peers are so much a part of each other's world—every day, our doctors connect with a colleague. With all that back and forth communication, you'd think it would be superb. However, different expectations, lack of time to consider how things are said, messages moving through staff instead of the doctor, and sometimes a little "he said, she said" have taken the glow off of peer-to-peer communication. The physician relations rep has a wonderful opportunity to provide some structure that may ensure connections are made, gaps are filled, and expectations are clearly defined. Formalize these elements within your program to support solid connections with the different types of physicians who refer within your medical staff.

Even with more methods and more real-time connectivity, there is a need to personalize the communication, to listen to the needs of our doctors, and ensure our communication with them meets their needs and ours. So, did I say, Game on? Know this: Nobody is better in this space than you are.

Summary

Physician relations reps need to seize the moment; be the choir director here. It requires confidence. You have to know the music, and you need to be in sync with what the audience wants to hear.

Physicians have clearly shared what they want to hear throughout the surveys we conducted. Now the opportunity exists to link those survey findings with the messages of the organization and to put it to your own voice.

C O N C L U S I O N

"Effective questioning brings insight, which fuels curiosity,
which cultivates wisdom."
—*Chip Bell*

The survey provided a wonderful perspective into the expectations of physicians, from their peer group, from organizational leaders, and from marketing and physician relations staffs. As a result, some perspectives and strategies may change within your organization. Or, at minimum, it may push the internal team to ask more questions before assuming that they know an answer.

After reviewing the data, one is more likely to consider messages and how they're delivered from the perspective of the doctor. Rather than one-size-fits-all communication tactics, consider who needs to hear the message. Four themes were evident throughout the survey findings.

1. **Learn from listening.** A wise doctor once shared with me, "If you listen long enough to the patient, they will give you the diagnosis." That premise is the same with most every audience. There's an opportunity to ask better questions and to really listen to the reply. Don't ask if you don't want to hear the reply. Listen with an open mind to the possibilities. Demonstrate you listened by communicating the response in an actionable way. The starting point is good dialogue with minds open and ears engaged.

2. **Ask and confirm, don't assume.** Assumptions and old baggage slow innovation and damage communication. The survey demonstrated that physicians want to be heard, so take the time to ask your doctors about topics of interest. This is a national survey. If you question whether some of the answers would hold true for your medical staff, ask them. It is human nature to enjoy being asked and offering opinions. If done in the right way, the organization can create a reliable pipeline to the thoughts and wishes of the medical staff.

3. **Flex the tools.** Marketers are immersed in discussions about the challenges of both cross-generational and cross-specialty communication vehicles. This is in play in all areas of communication with the medical staff. Whether it is one physician providing patient care input to another or a media tool to promote the practice, there is movement toward social media tools, but the audience is not all there yet. In the near term, successful communication with our doctors will use multiple methods, multiple times.

4. **Integrate communication into business and relationship strategies.** Real conversations about what doctors want to hear and what hospitals want to learn may not just happen in a hallway or in one of those spur-of-the-moment conversations. A real take-away from the survey is that there is a need to invest in communication. In these changing times, communication with the medical staff will be vital to creating better systems of care. Good communication pathways need to exist at every level of the organization and, likely, they will not occur without attention and effort.

NEW MODEL OF DIALOGUE

"While the survey results appropriately reference critical issues such as employment opportunities, quality, and practice support, my experience suggests that improved communications is a foundational element on which to build all of the other attributes. In fact, I believe classifying the issue as 'communications' is even too narrow in terms of defining language," says Jeff Cowart, senior vice president, growth and sales at Baptist Health System in San Antonio, TX.

Successful healthcare and hospital systems of the future will embrace physician engagement as stakeholders as the better model, he says. "Viewing physicians as stakeholders in health delivery and wellness for the community changes the nature of how and what needs to be communicated. Engaging or enrolling physicians as true stakeholders and as meaningful collaborators in the place of community trust that the hospital or healthcare system holds in the community is essential for success."

The stakeholder-engagement framework creates the promise of a new model of dialogue between the healthcare provider and the physician, explains Cowart. "Engagement promotes a higher level of surfacing and tracking physician dissatisfiers and acceleration of operational solutions. This framework, of a new model of communications, creates potential for such issues as employment to be addressed—not just as business deals, but as true partnerships in community service and relationships. Discussions of quality improvements can be elevated from checklists and protocols to a higher level of commitment to a shared noble mission."

What's Your Game Plan?

Do you step back, consider the contents of this book, and then throw yourself into the need of the moment? Do you test the survey results with members of your medical staff, just to make certain it is really true? Do you digress to remembering all the communication that you did well with limited response from the physicians and decide nothing will work?

That's last year's game. A better course of action today would be to vow to screen better and get communication to a more consistent and relevant level, find ways to gather a better sense of your physicians' needs as a part of the decision-making process, and use communication to reach out to physicians and say, "We'd welcome the chance to be in the game with you."

We asked what doctors wanted to hear because it is an important building block to strengthening the relationship with them. Now is your opportunity to use what we've learned.

About the Survey

The survey tool was designed with input from experts in each of the four areas addressed: marketing, leadership, peer-to-peer relations, and physician relations. The decision was made to fine-tune the questionnaire limiting the number of questions to ensure the survey was brief and easy for physicians to complete. Two survey tools were administered to keep the number of questions asked of any physician to a minimum. Some questions were included in both tools, whereas others appeared in only one of the surveys.

The survey was administered in December 2010 and January 2011. Several methods were used to gain response. A nationwide network of physician relations representatives was responsible for distributing the survey and collecting responses from physicians to ensure broad coverage and an adequate response rate. The representatives either interviewed doctors or e-mailed the survey tool to physicians in their market and on their medical staff. This list was further supplemented by a handful of personal contacts with physicians across the country.

Data analysis

A total of 190 interviews with physicians were completed using the techniques described here. Upon completion of the survey, the data were cleaned, verified, and tabulated in accordance with market research industry standards. Open-ended responses, where appropriate, were categorically coded for inclusion in the tabulated data tables. Data tables were created to show total responses as well as key demographic and geographic variables.

Response profile

The survey methodology provided excellent geographic coverage, with respondents representing approximately 26 states and more than 75 cities and communities across the country. Respondents included 24 clinical specialties spread across primary care and a number of medical and surgical specialties. In total, 56% of respondents were identified as primary care physicians, 38% were involved in the delivery of specialty care (i.e., medical, surgical, or hospital-based), and the remaining 6% were classified as other.

The age distribution of respondents was dominated by those in the 35 to 54 age range, although both older and younger groups were also represented in the sample (see Figure A.1).

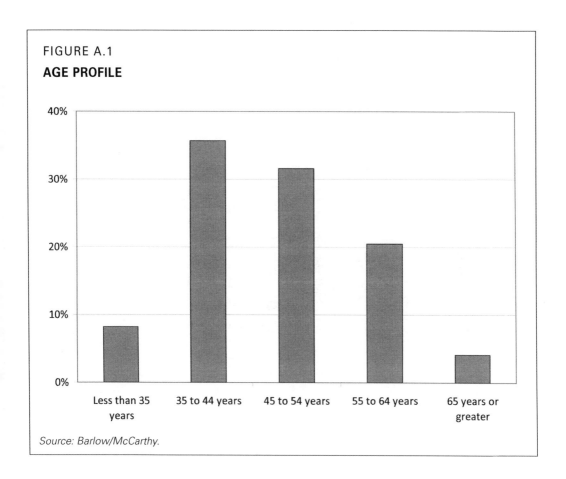

FIGURE A.1
AGE PROFILE

Source: Barlow/McCarthy.

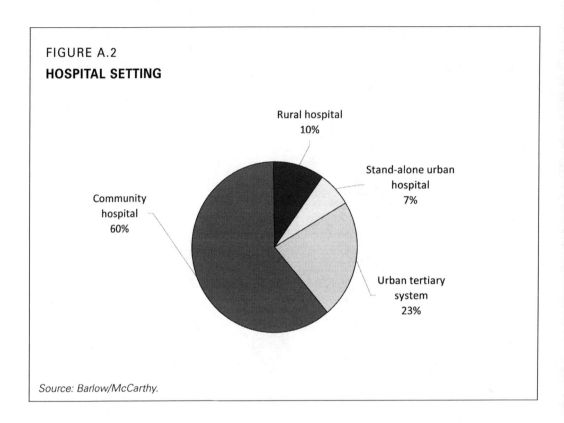

FIGURE A.2
HOSPITAL SETTING

Rural hospital
10%

Stand-alone urban
hospital
7%

Community
hospital
60%

Urban tertiary
system
23%

Source: Barlow/McCarthy.

Respondents covered the full range of hospital and practice settings. The majority of respondents identified the setting where they primarily practiced or referred most of their patients as a community-based hospital (61%), although the sample also included urban stand-alone facilities and tertiary centers as well as rural hospitals. Practice settings were also spread across the spectrum, including solo, small, and large single-specialty practices; multispecialty groups; and hospital-based practices (see Figures A.2 and A.3).

FIGURE A.3

PRACTICE SETTING

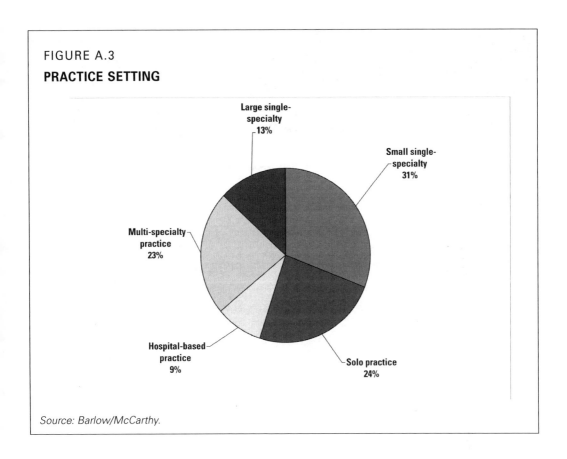

Large single-specialty
13%

Small single-specialty
31%

Multi-specialty
practice
23%

Hospital-based
practice
9%

Solo practice
24%

Source: Barlow/McCarthy.

FREE HEALTHCARE COMPLIANCE AND MANAGEMENT RESOURCES!

Need to control expenses yet stay current with critical issues?

Get timely help with FREE e-mail newsletters from HCPro, Inc., the leader in healthcare compliance education. Offering numerous free electronic publications covering a wide variety of essential topics, you'll find just the right e-newsletter to help you stay current, informed, and effective. All you have to do is sign up!

With your FREE subscriptions, you'll also receive the following:

- Timely information, to be read when convenient with your schedule
- Expert analysis you can count on
- Focused and relevant commentary
- Tips to make your daily tasks easier

And here's the best part: There's no further obligation—just a complimentary resource to help you get through your daily challenges.

It's easy. Visit *www.hcmarketplace.com/free/e-newsletters* to register for as many free e-newsletters as you'd like, and let us do the rest.

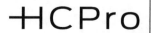

HCPro | Insight for healthcare compliance and management